Stop Spilling Your Soup!

THE COMPLETE ESSENTIAL TREMOR SOLUTION

Darlene A Mayo MD FAANS

ACKNOWLEDGMENTS

To God my Father and King, who created me in His perfect image, to Jesus Christ, my Lord and Savior, who calls me worthy even though I am a sinner, to the Holy Spirit, who guides me daily in all I do, I give You all the glory for what is created and written in this book. You gave me life, You give me breath. You save a place for me in heaven. You give me inspiration to write and lead people to the truth. You comfort me and You give me strength to do the work You have called me to do. Without You I am nothing and this work would not be possible.

Thank You.

To my loving husband, Shawn, you are my rock here on this earth. Your support, your passion for my happiness, your love, and your patience with me are beyond compare. You comfort me and encourage me when I think I can't. You are right there telling me that I can. You direct my eyes back to God and back to my purpose.

Thank You.

To Sylvie McCracken, my mentor in the writing of this book, you gave me the tools I needed to create this book, among them the mindset tools that are so very powerful. You introduced me to a network of like minded colleagues who support and encourage each other in such positive ways.

Thank You.

To my many, many neurosurgical mentors who trained me, mentored me, and inspired me to write the words in this book: Dr. Mark Lee, Dr. Joseph Smith, Dr. Alim Louis Benabid, Dr. Bob Gross, Dr. Ed Benzel.

Thank You.

To the many, many others who helped me in the review, marketing and production of this book: Sapna Desai, Stacey Grainger, Puneesh Goyal, Mike McClure. Without your hard work and dedication this book would not be as well written, as powerful, and as beautiful as it is.

Thank You.

DISCLAIMER: THIS BOOK DOES NOT PROVIDE MEDICAL ADVICE

TABLE OF CONTENTS

SECTION 2: AT HOME TREATMENTS

SECTION 3: MEDICAL AND SURGICAL OPTIONS

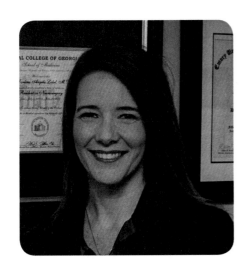

WHO I AM

My name is Darlene Mayo (née Lobel). I am a board-certified neurosurgeon who began practicing in 2007. I am trained and certified to practice all aspects of neurosurgery. The patients I have spent the most time treating over the last 10 years are much like many of you—they are people with tremors who want to know why they shake and how they can stop shaking.

I have known I wanted to be a doctor ever since I can remember, and I decided to become a neurosurgeon when I was in college. I had "shadowed" different doctors to see what their day-to-day lives were like. I looked into pediatrics, general surgery, and obstetrics. But the moment I walked into the operating room of Dr. Blaine Nashold and saw a living brain, I knew. That was it.

I love that the brain is so complex and that we know so little about it. I love that I could spend my whole life researching and practicing and never figure out all of the brain's intricacies. I think one of the things I love most about the brain is its possibilities. With so much unknown, anything is possible. I believe we have barely tapped into the power and capabilities of the brain. One of my goals in life is to learn how to use the brain to its fullest potential and to teach others how to do the same.

I spent 10 years in clinical practice at some of the top hospitals in the country helping people the best way I knew how—by sharing my medical knowledge, helping them develop the best plans for their treatment, and operating when I thought it would benefit them. I love this part of my career, because I have been able to see in an instant how life changing treatment such as deep brain stimulation can be.

I also have dedicated myself to researching new and better ways to treat patients with tremors and to helping patients make the best decisions for their medical treatment. I had the privilege and honor of working with Dr. Alim Louis Benabid in France, at one of the top research facilities in the world, for a couple of years. Dr. Benabid discovered the use of deep brain stimulation as a treatment for tremors due to essential tremor and Parkinson's disease, and he continues to pioneer many other innovations in medicine and scientific research to this day.

Furthermore, I am a teacher. I love sharing my knowledge with patients and doctors-in-training. I believe knowledge should be shared so that the next generation can be even better equipped than we are to challenge the limits of science and find cures for diseases and conditions. There are very few things to which I can compare the joy of seeing people—from medical students and neurosurgery residents (doctors-in-training) to those with limited or no medical knowledge—understand something new about the marvels of the brain.

So why did I write this book? Well, that is actually a very interesting story. I have always chosen to live my life by having faith in God and following His lead. About two years ago, I felt led to open my home to two foster children. That in turn led me to some significant realizations. First, raising children as a single mother makes brain surgery seem like a walk in the park! Seriously, though, these children are truly the joys and lights of my life, and they help me to grow in my faith daily. Along these lines, I realized that as much as I loved practicing neurosurgery, there was so much more that I could offer and learn. I began to view my calling in life in a broader way. I started to live my life walking day by day with God at my side and following His path for me, rather than the path that I had chosen on my own. So, over the last two years, my life has changed dramatically.

Almost a year ago, I was blessed to be able to adopt my children. God also brought my incredibly loving and amazing husband into my life. We were married a few months ago. With these beautiful changes in my life, I began to realize that my professional path must allow me to prioritize my family as well as my patients.

With great excitement, I decided to break from traditional neurosurgical practice. I began to consider new ways I could use my years of experience and medical knowledge to continue making an impact in the lives of my patients. Eventually, I was led to open a medical consulting business and to begin writing medical books for people looking for good quality information about available treatments. I have two goals in writing these books. First, it is important to me that people understand all of the treatment options out there, so part of this book focuses on non-medical and non-traditional therapies such as diet, exercise, and holistic treatments. I have worked hard to ensure there is reasonable scientific evidence to support the treatments included in this book.

Second, my patients often expressed that it was difficult to understand what they read about different treatments or what other doctors told them about their condition. I have always prioritized explaining complex medical procedures in easy-to-understand language. So, a large portion of this book is also dedicated to "translating" medical and surgical recommendations into clear and simple terms.

It is my hope that this book reaches and helps those of you who are looking for information but do not know where to start. I hope this book offers a beginning and helps you understand the basics about different ways tremor can be treated.

WHO THIS BOOK IS FOR

For people with tremor

I wrote this book primarily for those of you with essential tremor (ET) and tremors from other causes. I hope to help make your lives just a little better by giving you a guide, or handbook, if you will, of the best ideas I have studied, learned, and seen put into practice. Patients like you are the reason I went into medicine, and I have been blessed to be able to help hundreds of people with tremors through my career as a neurosurgeon. Now, I have come to realize that sharing my knowledge through this book carries the potential to reach infinitely more people with this condition.

For families of people with tremor

I also wrote this book for families of people with tremor. Sometimes we want so much to help a family member who is suffering that we settle for whatever resources we can find. I want to give you good quality information so you can help family members who shake understand the causes of their tremors and the different treatments that could help them.

For students, residents, and practicing physicians

I realize, too, that students of medicine, residents, and practicing physicians may find this book useful. This is meant to be understood by those without any medical knowledge, so it is not, say, a practitioner's how-to guide on managing patients with essential tremor. But perhaps this book will inspire a medical student to go into the field of neurosurgery or neurology and make an even greater impact in the lives of people with tremors. It is my hope that this book will also raise awareness of ET in the medical community and give doctors who do not generally treat this condition a resource for providing hope to their patients. I always find it difficult to tell a patient that I do not know what else I can do for them and that there is no one else to whom I can refer them. But it is so nice to be able to follow that up with this: there is more that **you** can do.

For researchers and innovators

Some of the concepts presented in this book, particularly the holistic approaches, are in the very early stages of discovery. They need further scientific research to find the best ways they can be used to help people with tremors. Perhaps something in this book will inspire a researcher to design a study to find answers or motivate an innovator to develop a new product to better control tremors.

HOW TO USE THIS BOOK

There are many ways to read this book. Some of you may be interested in reading it from start to finish. If you do, you will have a comprehensive understanding of the various holistic, medical, and surgical treatments available for tremors due to ET and some other causes.

Some of you may be interested in just one particular area. For example, maybe your doctor has recommended you have an MRI-guided focused ultrasound, and you want to know more about that. Or maybe you want to know about what you can do to help your tremors without ever setting foot in a doctor's office. The sections and chapters in this book are organized so that you can easily access the specific information you need. In addition, some chapters contain hyperlinks to other relevant sections of the book that you may find useful, as well.

This book is divided into five different sections. In Section 1, you will learn about the different causes of "tremors," or shaking. In Section 2, I describe various at-home treatments that you can do yourself to help reduce your tremors, from diet changes and easy exercises to herbal supplements you can take. Section 3 contains a wealth of information on the medical providers who can help figure out the cause of your tremors and recommend treatments. This section also describes in detail the different medical and surgical treatments available to help control tremors. Section 4 contains information on what are considered "alternative" medicine treatments, including acupuncture and other therapies, as well as information about the latest research studies on ET. Section 5 outlines strategies to help you make decisions about your medical care.

Keep in mind that it is unlikely you will significantly reduce your tremors with any one of these treatments alone. Most people will need to use a combination of different treatments to see the best results. Also remember that what works for one person may not work for another person.

Remember, too, that there is no cure for ET (at the time of the writing of this book). Many of the techniques I describe in this book can help make your tremors better. Most have documented scientific research behind them, and I tell you about these studies in each chapter. I also include helpful tips and tools that have not been studied formally but have anecdotally helped others.

Because updates to medical knowledge happen frequently, I keep a blog on my website (www.helpfortremors.com) that provides the most up-to-date information on new treatments and changes in current treatments. For news on major breakthroughs, you can subscribe to email updates through the website.

Please read through this book in the way you find most helpful, and feel free to email with any questions you may have.

Please sign up with your email to receive periodic updates about new treatments for essential tremor
https://drmayosbooks.com/contact

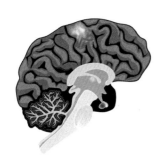
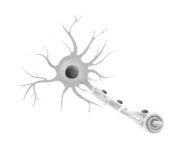
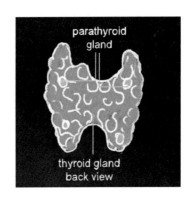

parathyroid
gland

thyroid gland
back view

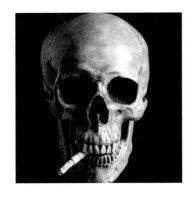
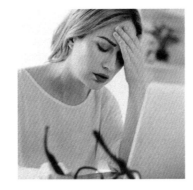
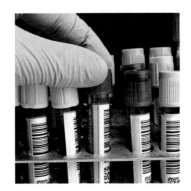

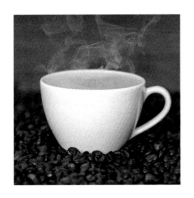
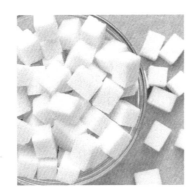
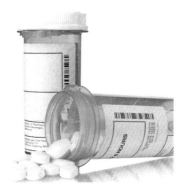

SECTION

1

WHY AM I SHAKING?

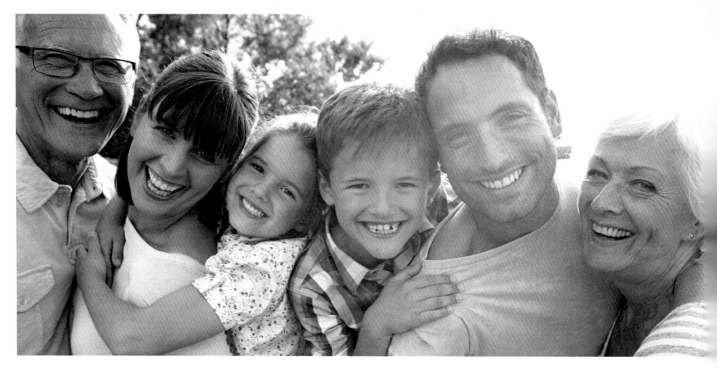

EVERYONE SHAKES

Seeing your own arm shake can be scary! "That isn't supposed to happen," you may think. Then you may decide to look on the internet, maybe using Google or the symptom checker on WebMD, to figure out what is wrong. Sometimes this can be helpful. But sometimes you may read things that are frightening. Remember that some information on the internet is of good quality, while other websites give you "half-truths," particularly where medical conditions are concerned. So how are you supposed to know where to look and what to do?

First, I will ask you to stop for a moment, take a deep breath in, and then breathe out slowly. Know that you are in the right place to find quality information that will likely help ease your fears. This book is based on years and years of my experience evaluating and treating patients who shake. In this section, I will tell you about the most common causes of shaking and the symptoms you may see with each of these conditions. You should also know that unless your doctor has told you that you have essential tremor or a similar disorder, there is a good chance that you do not have a medical condition that is causing you to shake.

Did you know that everyone has some tremor? It's true! Everybody shakes sometimes and to some degree. This type of tremor is known as "physiologic tremor." Physiologic tremor is a very fine shaking in your hands and fingers that comes and goes. In some people it is barely noticeable, while in others it can be quite obvious. You may see this tremor when you are sitting still, or when you are trying to do an activity, like eating or drinking. Usually, physiologic tremor causes shaking in both hands, although one hand may shake more than the other.[1] Researchers do not understand what causes this type of shaking, but they do know the kinds of things that make this "natural tremor" worse. These include caffeine, too much or too little sugar in your system, smoking, certain medicines, recreational drugs, alcohol, stress, and tired muscles. Interestingly, the things that make physiologic tremor worse often make tremors due to other causes worse, as well.

Caffeine

Caffeine is a substance found in coffee, some teas and soft drinks, and certain foods, such as chocolate. It is considered a stimulant, which means many people use it to be more alert in the mornings or during the day when they feel low on energy. Caffeine can have some positive effects on the brain, including enhancing your memory.[2] Recent research also shows that small amounts of caffeine over a period of time can reduce your risk of developing Parkinson's or Alzheimer's diseases.[3] However, caffeine, particularly in high amounts, can also have negative effects on the nervous system and can make tremors of any kind (physiologic or otherwise) much worse.[4]

» One way to reduce your tremors (due to any cause) may be to decrease your caffeine intake.

Sugar

There has been a lot of discussion in recent years about how harmful processed sugar (table sugar and added sugars in foods) can be to your body. Too much processed sugar can lead to everything from early heart disease and stroke to weight gain and diabetes.[5] There is even a link between sugar intake and the progression of certain cancers.[6,7]

Eating too much sugar causes problems with the way your body naturally processes sugar and turns it into "nutrients" you can use.[8] The chemical that controls the amount of sugar in your body (your "blood sugar") is called insulin. Insulin can be released in your body in really high amounts after you eat a lot of sugar. As a result, your blood sugar levels may first become very high (also known as hyperglycemia) and then very low (also known as hypoglycemia). When your blood sugar is very low, you can start to shake,[9] or the tremors you already have can become much worse. When blood sugar is critically low, you can even develop seizures.[10]

» Another way to reduce tremors may be to limit the amount of processed sugar you eat.

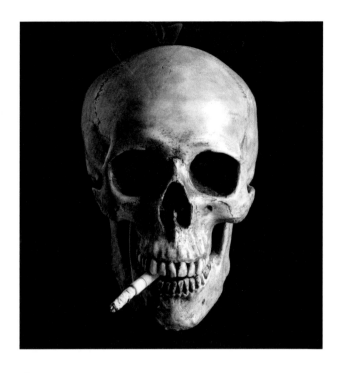

Smoking

Did you know that smoking cigarettes or using tobacco in other forms can cause you to shake?[11] Most people who smoke will tell you that one of the reasons they do it is to calm themselves down. However, studies have shown that nicotine is a stimulant and that smoking actually increases anxiety.[12] Further, research studies have found that smoking is harmful to many parts of your body, including your lungs, heart, and brain,[13] and also makes tremors worse.[11,14] Quitting smoking even for a day can help lessen tremors.[15]

Keep in mind that the first few days or weeks after you stop smoking, your body may go through "withdrawal" from nicotine (the main ingredient in cigarettes), which can make your tremors worse.[16] This effect should fade away the longer you go without smoking. You can find many resources on how to quit smoking on the website www.smokefree.gov, and there are many apps you can get for your smartphone that may be helpful. Also, your doctor can give you medicines to help you quit.

» Quitting smoking is another way you can slow down your tremors.

Medicines

Certain medicines that your doctor gives you can have side effects that cause tremors or make them worse. While the full list is very long, below are some of the most common medicines people take that can cause or worsen tremors.[17-24]

High blood pressure
- *Hydrochlorothiazide*
- *Losartan*

Asthma/breathing difficulty
- *Albuterol*
- *Theophylline*

Depression
- *Citalopram (common brand name: Celexa)*
- *Imipramine (Tofranil)*
- *Paroxetine (Paxil)*

Seizures
- *Valproate*

If you take any of these medicines, talk to your doctor about the possibility of switching to a different medicine to treat your condition. In some cases, it may safe to change medicines. In other cases, there may not be a different medicine that will help you as much. As with all medical decisions, you and your doctor will need to work together to understand the risks and benefits of switching medicines.

» Changing medicines may help reduce your tremors.

Recreational drugs

Certain recreational drugs can make your tremors worse. These include cocaine, methamphetamine, heroin, whippets, and ecstasy. In addition to causing many serious health problems, using these drugs can affect the chemicals in your brain and cause tremors.[25]

» To keep your tremors from getting worse, avoid taking recreational drugs.

ALCOHOL

The effects alcohol has on tremor are complex. In small, infrequent amounts (one or two glasses of wine every once in a while), alcohol can dramatically reduce your tremor.[25] But keep in mind that alcohol has side effects that include clouding your judgment and making it harder to control your muscles.[26] So, while drinking a couple glasses of wine may reduce your tremor, you will not be able to use this as a treatment all the time. For example, you would not want to drink before going to work or driving a car.

Further, the day after you drink, you may feel the effects of alcohol withdrawal, which can include worsened tremors.[25] Drinking alcohol frequently and in large amounts can also lead to addiction, which can cause many health problems including liver damage and even brain damage.[26] Brain damage from high amounts of alcohol intake over several years can increase tremors.[25,27] Currently, researchers are trying to develop a medicine made from a type of alcohol that would not cause the same side effects. See the chapter on **Research in Section 4** of this book to learn more about this.

If you think you may have a problem with drinking too much alcohol, please talk to your doctor. There are many resources available to help you stop drinking.

Having small amounts of alcohol on occasion may decrease your tremors, while drinking large amounts frequently can have serious negative effects on your health.

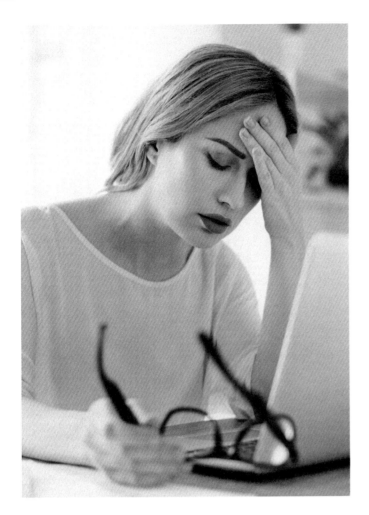

hands and knees may tremble. Sometimes your whole body may even shake.

Fortunately, there are many, many treatments that can lower your stress levels, such as meditation, yoga, massage, tai chi, acupuncture, and anti-anxiety medicines, to name a few. See the chapters "Activities that slow down tremors" in Section 2 and "Alternative treatments" in Section 4 for more information on ways these treatments can help reduce tremors.

» Lowering your stress levels is likely to slow down your tremors.

Tired muscles

Doing a lot of physical activity, or doing challenging exercises for even 5-10 minutes, puts strain on your muscles. Have you ever noticed that after you did something physically strenuous, like raking the yard or exercising with heavy weights, your arms or hands started to shake?

Researchers have found that when your muscles get fatigued, or tired, from straining with either a heavy weight for a few minutes or no weight for a long time, your brain sends a signal to your arms or legs that makes them shake.[30,31] Sometimes this shaking can last for a few minutes or even a few hours.[32] Tremor caused by muscle fatigue even affects surgeons! We learn ways to hold and support our arms and hands in order to decrease the tremor that happens after a few hours in surgery so that we can safely keep operating.

Even though your tremor may get worse just after you finish exercising, strengthening your muscles through exercise can help decrease your tremors in the long run. See Section 2 for more information on exercises you can try to help your tremors.

» Tired muscles can make your tremors worse, but long-term exercise can help slow down your tremors.

Stress

We all know what it is like to have stress in our lives. Stress from situations that are hard to deal with—from something minor like getting a traffic ticket, to something major like losing your job or having a family member die—causes not only emotional pain but also physical issues. While some stress can be helpful (such as nervousness about passing a test, which causes you to study), stress that never seems to go away can be very harmful to your health.

Stress causes changes to the chemicals in your body. When you feel stress, your body releases a chemical called cortisol.[28] High amounts of cortisol in your body can cause many problems, including damage to your heart and an increased chance of you getting infections.[29] Additionally, when you are stressed, your tremors get worse immediately. Think about when you feel nervous or afraid. Your

CHAPTER SUMMARY

The following tips may help to reduce "natural tremor" and tremor from other causes.

- *Avoid large amounts of caffeine*
- *Avoid processed sugar*
- *Stop smoking*
- *Talk to your doctor about changing medicines you take*
- *Avoid taking recreational drugs*
- *Avoid large amounts of alcohol over a long time*
- *Keep your stress levels low*
- *Exercise regularly*

REFERENCES

1. Lauk M, Köster B, Timmer J, Guschlbauer B, Deuschl G, Lücking CH. Side-to-side correlation of muscle activity in physiological and pathological human tremors. *Clin Neurophysiol.* 1999;110(10):1774-83.

2. Sherman SM, Buckley TP, Baena E, Ryan L. Caffeine enhances memory performance in young adults during their non-optimal time of day. *Front Psychol.* Nov 2016;7:1764.

3. Tellone E, Galtieri A, Russo A, Ficarra S. Protective effects of the caffeine against neurodegenerative diseases. *Curr Med Chem.* Oct 2017. doi: 10.2174/0929867324 666171009104040.

4. Humayun MU, Rader RS, Pieramici DJ, Awh CC, de Juan E Jr. Quantitative measurement of the effects of caffeine and propranolol on surgeon hand tremor. *Arch Ophthalmol.* 1997;115(3):371-4.

5. Johnson RK, Appel LJ, Brands M, et al. Dietary sugars intake and cardiovascular health: a scientific statement from the American Heart Association. *Circulation.* 2009;120(11):1011-20.

6. Warburg O. On the origin of cancer cells. *Science.* 1956;123:309–314.

7. Liao WC, Tu YK, Wu MS, Lin JT, Wang HP, Chien KL. Blood glucose concentration and risk of pancreatic cancer: systematic review and dose-response meta-analysis. *BMJ.* 2015;350:g7371.

8. Macdonald IA. A review of recent evidence relating to sugars, insulin resistance and diabetes. *Eur J Nutr.* 2016;55(Suppl 2):17–23.

9. Berlin I, Grimaldi A, Landault C, Cesselin F, Puech AJ. Suspected postprandial hypoglycemia is associated with beta-adrenergic hypersensitivity and emotional distress. *J Clin Endocrinol Metab.* 1994;79(5):1428-33.

10. Malouf R, Brust JC. Hypoglycemia: causes, neurological manifestations, and outcome. *Ann Neurol.* 1985;17(5):421-30.

11. Shiffman SM, Gritz ER, Maltese J, Lee MA, Schneider NG, Jarvik ME. Effects of cigarette smoking and oral nicotine on hand tremor. *Clin Pharmacol Ther.* 1983;33(6):800-5.

12. McDermott MS, Marteau TM, Hollands GJ, Hankins M, Aveyard P. Change in anxiety following successful and unsuccessful attempts at smoking cessation: cohort study. *Br J Psychiatry*. 2013;202(1):62-7.

13. Centers for Disease Control and Prevention. *How tobacco smoke causes disease: The biology and behavioral basis for smoking-attributable disease: A report of the Surgeon General*. Atlanta, GA: Centers for Disease Control and Prevention; 2010. Available from: www.ncbi.nlm.nih.gov/books/NBK53017.

14. G SB, Choi S, Krishnan J, K R. Cigarette smoke and related risk factors in neurological disorders: An update. *Biomed Pharmacother*. 2017;85:79-86.

15. Gilbert RM, Pope MA. Early effects of quitting smoking. *Psychopharmacology (Berl)*. 1982;78(2):121-7.

16. Mengesha J. 5 Things You Need to Know About Nicotine Withdrawal and Anxiety. Livestrong.com. https://www.livestrong.com/article/204934-how-do-i-reduce-jitters-from-quitting-smoking. Published August 24, 2017.

17. Drugs.com. Hydrochlorothiazide Side Effects. https://www.drugs.com/sfx/hydrochlorothiazide-side-effects.html.

18. Drugs.com. Losartan Side Effects. https://www.drugs.com/sfx/losartan-side-effects.html.

19. Drugs.com. Albuterol Side Effects. https://www.drugs.com/sfx/albuterol-side-effects.html.

20. Drugs.com. Theophylline Side Effects. https://www.drugs.com/sfx/theophylline-side-effects.html.

21. Drugs.com. Citalopram Side Effects. https://www.drugs.com/sfx/citalopram-side-effects.html.

22. Drugs.com. Tofranil-PM Side Effects. https://www.drugs.com/sfx/tofranil-pm-side-effects.html.

23. Drugs.com. Paxil Side Effects. https://www.drugs.com/sfx/paxil-side-effects.html.

24. Drugs.com. Valproate Sodium Side Effects. https://www.drugs.com/sfx/valproate-sodium-side-effects.html.

25. Deik A, Saunders-Pullman R, San Luciano M. Substances of abuse and movement disorders: complex interactions and comorbidities. *Curr Drug Abuse Rev*. 2012; 5(3): 243–253.

26. Liang J, Olsen RW. Alcohol use disorders and current pharmacological therapies: the role of GABA receptors. *Acta Pharmacol Sin*. 2014;35(8):981–993.

27. Silva D, Matias C, Bourne S, Nagel S, Machado A, Lobel D. Effects of chronic alcohol consumption on long-term outcomes of thalamic deep brain stimulation for essential tremor. *J Clin Neurosci*. 2016;31:142-6.

28. van Eck M; Berkhof H; Nicolson N, Sulon J. The effects of perceived stress, traits, mood states, and stressful daily events on salivary cortisol. *Psychosom Med*. 1996;58(5):447-458.

29. Schneiderman N, Ironson G, Siegel SD. Stress and health: psychological, behavioral, and biological determinants. *Annu Rev Clin Psychol*. 2005;1:607-628.

30. Viitasalo JT, Gajewski J. Effects of strength training-induced fatigue on tremor spectrum in elbow flexion. *Hum Mov Sci*. 1994; 13(1):129-141.

31. Morrison S, Kavanagh J, Obst SJ, Irwin J, Haseler LJ. The effects of unilateral muscle fatigue on bilateral physiological tremor. *Exp Brain Res*. 2005;167(4):609–621.

32. Dartnall TJ, Nordstrom MA, Semmler JG. Motor unit synchronization is increased in biceps brachii after exercise-induced damage to elbow flexor muscles. *J Neurophys*. 2008;99(2):1008-1019.

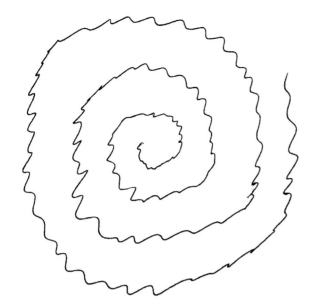

ESSENTIAL TREMOR

WHAT IT IS

Essential tremor, or ET, is the most common cause of shaking in adults (other than "natural" or "physiologic" tremor) and is the most common "movement disorder." You may have also heard ET called "benign essential tremor" (BET). This is an older term that was used because essential tremor was not considered a disease and was considered to be a "benign," or harmless, issue. Recently, doctors have begun to realize the many ways ET can negatively impact someone's life, so most doctors no longer use the word "benign" to describe ET.

Your arms and hands may seem to shake in a rhythm in ET, and the tremor often occurs on both sides of the body.[1] In some cases, ET may cause one side of your body to shake more than the other.[2] Sometimes tremor may be stronger in your dominant hand (the one you use to write or do most tasks); however, sometimes it is worse in your other hand. It is possible to have tremor in only one arm or hand or even in one finger. Some people only have tremors when doing very specific activities, such as playing violin.[3] ET can also cause your head or voice to shake. Tremors often get worse over time and can keep you from doing the things you want to do.[4]

One interesting fact about ET is that the shaking usually happens when you are trying to do a specific activity, like eating, drinking, writing, using a computer or cell phone, or trying to turn a key in a lock. This is called an "action tremor." You can also have "postural tremor," which means your arms shake when you hold them out in front of you. It is very uncommon to shake when you are sitting still, unless your tremor is very severe.[1,2] Many people with ET also have other issues, such as depression (sadness) or anxiety (nervousness).[2] Sometimes the anxiety could be so serious that you do not want to go out in public. It is very common to feel embarrassed about your shaking. Sometimes others may assume that you are shaking from drinking too much or other reasons, rather than understanding that you have a medical condition.

How common is ET?

ET affects approximately 2.2 to 6 percent of the population in the US,[1,5] which means between 2 and 6 out of every 100 people have ET. Interestingly, many researchers believe these estimates are too low. Some doctors are not trained to recognize the signs and symptoms of ET,[6] and people often do not realize their shaking could be caused by ET.[7] Others may think that shaking is normal, particularly as people get older. This thought process is very common in family members of those who have tremor.

With the introduction of "Essential Tremor Awareness Month" each March and other initiatives by organizations such as the International Essential Tremor Foundation (IETF) and National Tremor Foundation (NTF), ET is becoming more widely recognized. People are starting to learn more about tremors and that there is help for people with ET. As this information and awareness keeps spreading, and more people see their doctors about ET, we may find that ET is more common than we think.

Darlene A Mayo MD FAANS   **STOP SPILLING YOUR SOUP!   The Complete Essential Tremor Solution**

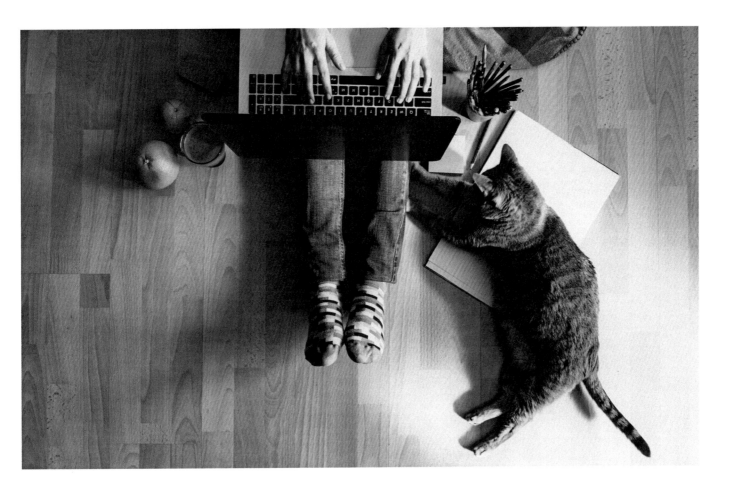

At what age do most people get ET?

ET can affect people at any age. Doctors most commonly "diagnose," or recognize, ET in people in their 50s. However, many people notice shaking even in their teenage years or earlier in childhood.[8,9] Often the shaking does not bother them much or keep them from doing regular tasks until they get older. This is when they finally see a doctor to find out what is causing their shaking.

My father has ET. How likely am I to get it?

ET runs in families. If you have a parent who has ET, you generally have a 50/50 chance of also getting ET.[1,10] About half of the people who have ET do not have a family member with the condition.

What causes ET?

It is not known exactly what causes ET. Some research suggests that, in ET, a chemical in the brain called GABA either is not made in the right amount or does not work properly.[11] Researchers are also looking for the gene or genes that may be responsible for ET.

Is there a cure for ET?

There is no known cure for ET. However, the good news is that there are MANY things that you can do to slow down or stop your shaking!

How do I know if I have ET?

Doctors will usually be able to tell you if you have ET simply by getting information from you and examining you in their office. Your doctor may order a special x-ray, called an MRI, to make sure you don't have another reason for shaking. Sometimes, he or she may order other tests, called PET and SPECT scans, to help them figure out if your tremor is caused by ET or Parkinson's disease. These x-rays should be normal in people with ET.

Facts about ET

- *It is the most common cause of shaking in adults*
- *It can happen at any age*
- *It runs in families*
- *We don't know exactly what causes it*
- *There is no cure*
- *Your doctor can usually tell if you have it without special tests*
- *There are MANY treatments available*

REFERENCES

1. Crawford P, Zimmerman EE. Differentiation and diagnosis of tremor. *Am Fam Physician*. 2011;83(6):697-702.

2. Sharma S, Pandey S. Approach to a tremor patient. *Ann Indian Acad Neurol*. 2016;19(4):433–443.

3. Lee A, Furuya S, and Altenmuller E. Epidemiology and treatment of 23 musicians with task specific tremor. *J Clin Mov Disord*. 2014;1:5.

4. Gutierrez J, Park J, Badejo O, Louis ED. Worse and worse and worse: essential tremor patients' longitudinal perspectives on their condition. *Front Neurol*. 2016;7:175.

5. Louis ED, and Ottman R. How many people in the USA have essential tremor? Deriving a population estimate based on epidemiological data. *Tremor Other Hyperkinet Mov*. 2014;4:259.

6. Lobel DA, Kahn M, Rosen CL, Pilitsis JG. Medical student education in neurosurgery: optional or essential? *Teach Learn Med*. 2015;27(2):201-4.

7. Rajput AH, Rajput A. Medical treatment of essential tremor. *J Cent Nerv Syst Dis*. 2014;6:29-39.

8. Elias WJ, Shah BB. Tremor. *JAMA*. 2014;311(9):948-954.

9. National Institute of Neurological Disorders and Stroke. Tremor fact sheet. http://www.ninds.nih.gov/Disorders/Patient-Caregiver-Education/Fact-Sheets/Tremor-Fact-Sheet. Published May 2017. Updated July 12, 2017.

10. International Essential Tremor Foundation. Facts about essential tremor. https://www.essentialtremor.org/wp-content/uploads/2013/07/FactSheet012013.pdf. Published January 2013.

11. Gironell A. The GABA hypothesis in essential tremor: lights and shadows. *Tremor Other Hyperkinet Mov (N Y)*. 2014;4:254

There are many different conditions that can cause you to shake. While much of this book focuses one of the most common causes of shaking, essential tremor (ET), this chapter covers other reasons you may shake. This is not a complete list but rather a general overview of the more common issues that can cause tremor. Among these are Parkinson's disease (PD), thyroid problems, multiple sclerosis (MS), stroke, brain tumors, and vitamin deficiencies. When reading through the symptoms of each condition, remember that not everyone will have all of the symptoms described, and others may have symptoms that are not listed.

PARKINSON'S DISEASE

WHAT IT IS

Parkinson's disease, or PD, is a very common movement disorder that often causes shaking. Unlike ET, PD always starts on one side of your body. Even if PD eventually affects both sides, one side will almost always be worse.[1] Also unlike ET, if you have PD you will shake mostly while you are sitting still. This is called a "resting tremor." You may also shake while trying to do things like eat and write.[2] **So, many of the techniques described in this book will still be useful to you if you have PD.**

In addition to shaking, PD also causes other problems. Very commonly, you will have stiffness in your arms and legs, be slow to move, and may even have episodes of "freezing," in which you stop while walking and cannot take another step for a period of time. You may also have problems with sleep, swallowing, or your bladder, among other issues. The problems caused by PD tend to get worse over time.[1]

HOW COMMON IS IT?

You are much less likely to develop PD than you are to have ET. The most recent estimates suggest that only 0.15 to 0.3 percent of people in the US have PD.[3] This means about 2 to 3 out of every 1000 people have PD (while 2 to 6 out of every 100 people have ET). Interestingly, some studies show that you are more likely to get ET if you have PD, and vice versa. This may be related to genetics and is being further studied.[4]

AT WHAT AGE DO MOST PEOPLE GET IT?

Doctors usually first notice PD in people in their 50s or 60s. There are some people with PD who show signs of the disease as early as their 30s or 40s. Michael J. Fox is a good example of someone who developed "early onset" PD.[5]

MY FATHER HAS PD. HOW LIKELY AM I TO GET IT?

PD does run in some families; however, if you have a relative with PD, you only have about a 15 percent chance of getting the disorder.[6] Most people who get PD do not have any other family members with the disease.

WHAT CAUSES IT?

PD happens when your brain does not make enough of a certain brain chemical called "dopamine." Dopamine is made by cells in the base of the brain, in an area called the "substantia nigra." If about 70 percent of these cells stop making dopamine, you will start showing signs of PD.[1] Researchers do not really understand what causes these cells to stop making dopamine, but they do know that certain genes are not normal in some people with PD.[6]

IS THERE A CURE?

There is no known cure for PD. As with ET, there are many things you can do to help decrease your tremors and some of the other medical problems caused by PD. Typically, treatments include medicines as well as many of the therapies described in this book.

HOW DO I KNOW IF I HAVE IT?

Doctors will often be able to tell you if you have PD simply by getting information from you and examining you in their office. There are also special x-rays, called PET and SPECT scans, that doctors sometimes use to help them figure out whether you have PD.[7]

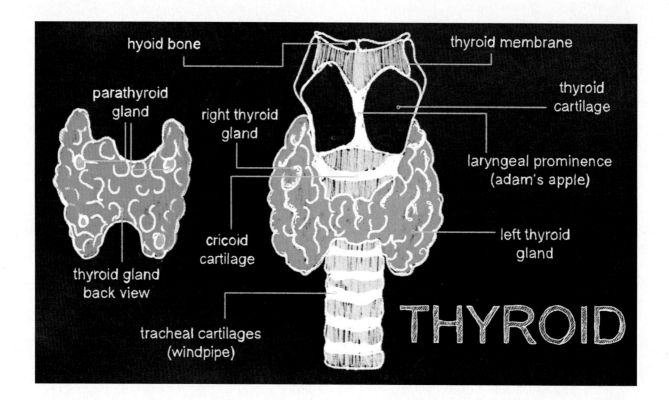

hyoid bone

thyroid membrane

parathyroid gland

right thyroid gland

thyroid cartilage

laryngeal prominence (adam's apple)

cricoid cartilage

left thyroid gland

thyroid gland back view

tracheal cartilages (windpipe)

THYROID

HYPERTHYROIDISM

What it is

Hyperthyroidism is a problem with your thyroid gland, which is a small gland located in the front of your neck. This gland produces a hormone that affects your energy levels, weight, skin, and brain, among many other things. When your thyroid hormone levels get too high, it can cause you to have tremors.[8] Also, if you take too much of a medicine to treat low thyroid levels, you can have tremors as well.[9] Typically, if you have tremors caused by thyroid problems, they will occur while you are performing a movement (intention tremor) and will affect both arms and both legs equally.[8]

How common is it?

About one percent of people in the US are estimated to have hyperthyroidism.[10]

At what age do most people get it?

Hyperthyroidism can happen at any age.[11]

What causes it?

There are many different causes of hyperthyroidism. These include problems with the thyroid gland itself, problems with the brain, and other issues.[11]

Is there a cure?

Yes. Hyperthyroidism is treated differently depending on what causes it. You may need medicines and possibly surgery. Some people need to keep taking medicines throughout their lives to keep their thyroid hormone levels normal. Once your thyroid hormone levels return to normal, your tremors will likely stop.[8]

How do I know if I have it?

Your doctor can tell you if you have hyperthyroidism by doing a blood test.

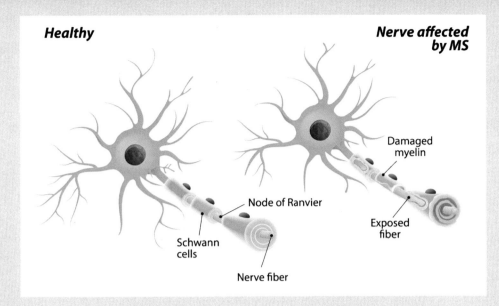

Healthy   *Nerve affected by MS*

Damaged myelin

Node of Ranvier

Exposed fiber

Schwann cells

Nerve fiber

WHAT IT IS

Multiple sclerosis, or MS, is a condition that causes damage to your brain and spinal cord.

In addition to tremors, MS can cause many issues, including tingling, numbness, or weakness in your arms or legs and problems with your vision.[12] The tremors you have with MS may cause your arms, legs, head, or voice to shake, much like you would see with ET. Tremor caused by MS will most commonly happen when you are performing a movement and may be on one side of the body or both.[13]

HOW COMMON IS IT?

MS is a somewhat rare disease, affecting around 2 out of every 1000 people. It is more common in women and people who live in the Northern hemisphere.[14,15]

AT WHAT AGE DO MOST PEOPLE GET IT?

MS usually first shows up in young adults between the ages of 20 and 40.[12]

WHAT CAUSES IT?

We do not fully understand what causes MS. We do know that in MS your immune system (the part of your body that helps fight infections) does not work properly. Some researchers think genes may play a role, while others think MS may be related to smoking cigarettes or not having enough vitamin D in your body.[16]

IS THERE A CURE FOR IT?

There is no cure for MS at this time. You can use medicines, physical therapy, and alternative medicine techniques to help control your symptoms. If you have tremor caused by MS, it may get better when you treat your MS.[17]

HOW DO I KNOW IF I HAVE IT?

Your doctor can tell if you have MS by doing a test called a spinal tap and getting a special x-ray of your brain and spinal cord called an MRI.[16]

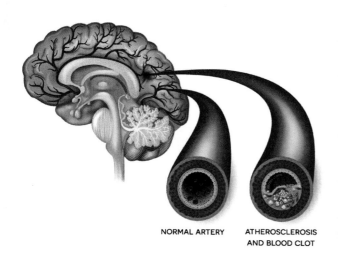

NORMAL ARTERY   ATHEROSCLEROSIS
AND BLOOD CLOT

STROKE

What it is

A stroke, or "brain attack," causes damage to your brain when an artery (which carries blood to the brain) gets blocked or when there is bleeding in your brain. A stroke usually affects one part of the brain. Depending on the part of your brain affected, you will have different symptoms. Strokes almost always cause problems that come on quickly. This is one of the reasons that the catch phrase "Act FAST" is used to recognize the signs of a stroke.[18]

Face: Try to smile—can you only smile with half of your face?

Arms: Lift both your arms (or legs)—do you have trouble lifting one? Does one fall back down?

Speech: Try to say something—is it hard to speak? Are you slurring your words?

Time: If you see any of these signs, call 911 immediately.

A stroke often suddenly makes one side of your body weak, making it difficult or impossible to use your arm or leg. A stroke can also make you have trouble speaking. Some, but not all, strokes cause tremor. This tremor will almost always be on only one side of your body. Strokes cause different kinds of tremor depending on whether they affect the middle of your brain (midbrain) or the back (cerebellum). A midbrain stroke will cause your hand to shake at rest or when your arm is held out in front of you. A cerebellar stroke will make you shake mainly while you are trying to perform a movement.[13] Keep in mind that in rare cases, you could have a small stroke without showing any signs other than tremor.

How common is it?

About 3 out of every 100 people will have a stroke in their lifetime. In older adults, that number is much higher. After the age of 55, one out of every five women and one out of every six men will have a stroke. Stroke is the fifth most common cause of death in the US and the second most common worldwide.[19]

At what age do most people get it?

As mentioned above, strokes are much more common after the age of 55. However, a stroke can occur at any age.

What causes it?

There are many things that can increase your chances of having a stroke. These include cigarette smoking, a diet high in fats and cholesterol, stress, high blood pressure, not exercising, and health issues such as diabetes, kidney problems, and heart problems.[19]

Is there a cure?

It is very important that you call 911 immediately if you think you are having a stroke. Sometimes they will tell you to go to the nearest emergency room so you can be evaluated and treated. Other times they may be able to send you a "mobile stroke unit," which is like a special ambulance that handles strokes.

Sometimes the effects of a stroke can be reversed. Once a stroke has happened, there is a small window of time (less than six hours) to have this type treatment, which involves doctors doing a procedure to remove a blood clot from your artery (thrombectomy) and/or giving you medicines to help the blood clot dissolve (thrombolysis). Not everyone who has a stroke can have this treatment. For example, if you are already taking a medicine to thin your blood, or if the type of stroke you have is one that causes bleeding in the brain, it would not be safe to have this procedure.

Know that even if you can't have the "reversal" procedure, you can still get treatment after a stroke. With physical therapy, speech therapy, and/or medicines to help keep your blood thin, you may be able to recover function within one year after a stroke.[20,21] If you have tremor caused by a stroke, it may or may not get better as you recover.

How do I know if I have it?

A special x-ray called a CT or an MRI will help your doctor know whether you have had a stroke.

BRAIN TUMOR

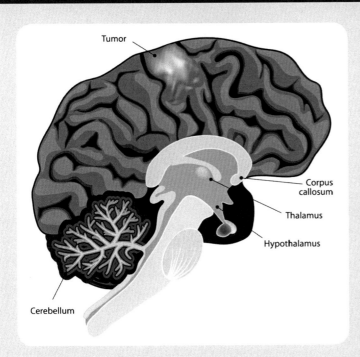

Tumor
Corpus callosum
Thalamus
Hypothalamus
Cerebellum

WHAT IT IS

A brain tumor is a mass that forms in the brain because either brain cells are growing abnormally or a cancer somewhere else in the body has traveled (metastasized) to the brain. Much like a stroke, a brain tumor can form in many different parts of the brain. Depending on the spot in which the tumor grows, you can have different symptoms, including a weak arm or leg, trouble speaking,

or difficulty walking. The weakness you get from a brain tumor is usually mild at first. It may just seem like you are getting clumsy and dropping things. This is different from the weakness you would feel with a stroke, which would cause you to lose total control of your arm or leg. Also, unlike with a stroke, problems due to a brain tumor usually happen very slowly over time. The most common sign people first have is a seizure.[22] There are many different types of seizures—some may cause you to stare off into space for a few seconds or minutes, while others may cause you to fall to the ground, shake violently, and pass out.

Sometimes people with brain tumors have headaches, but before you start worrying that your occasional headache means you have a brain tumor, please read this next sentence. **Headaches caused by brain tumors have very specific signs and you will almost always have more problems than just a headache.** A headache from a brain tumor is usually worse in the morning, bothers you almost every day, and often keeps getting worse day by day. The headache is often in the front of your head and worse on one side of your head. You may also feel sick to your stomach and throw up.[23] A headache caused by a brain tumor is different from a migraine, which often gets better after you lie down and rest.[24] Lastly, along with the headache you usually will have weakness in your arm or leg or trouble speaking.

Brain tumors can also cause tremors. Just like with stroke, if you have a tumor in the back of your brain (cerebellum), your tremor will mainly happen when you are trying to do an activity. You can also have resting tremors if your tumor is near the top or middle of your brain. Brain tumors almost always cause tremors only on one side of the body.[25]

HOW COMMON IS IT?

Brain tumors are extremely rare, occurring in only 2 or 3 people out of every 100,000. Women are more likely to have benign (non-cancerous) tumors, while men are more likely to have cancerous tumors.[26] Although brain tumors are rare in general and a rare cause of tremors, I chose to include them in this chapter because they are something that people often worry about.

AT WHAT AGE DO MOST PEOPLE GET IT?

Brain tumors can happen to people of all ages, from newborn babies to the very old. Some tumors are more common in different age groups. The most common type of primary brain tumor (not metastatic), glioma, happens often in people in their 70s and 80s, although sometimes it can affect people in their 30s and 40s as well.[27]

WHAT CAUSES IT?

We do not fully understand what causes most brain tumors. Some tumors are thought to be caused by problems in your genes, while others are thought to be caused by things in the environment, such as radiation, nuclear power plants, lead or other dangerous chemicals, and cigarette smoke. All of these things have all been linked to higher rates of brain tumors. The discussion about whether cell phone use can cause tumors is still hotly debated.[26]

IS THERE A CURE?

It depends. Some brain tumors can be "cured" by surgery or special types of radiation. These types of tumors are considered "benign." We usually refer to this cure as "remission," because a benign tumor can sometimes come back even after you have had surgery to remove all of it. Some tumors cannot be completely removed or cannot be removed at all if they are in a part of your brain that controls vital functions (like breathing, heartbeat, consciousness, etc.). Also, sometimes you will have chemotherapy (medicines) and/or different types of radiation treatment for tumors. Keep in mind that certain chemotherapy medicines can also cause tremors.[28]

HOW DO I KNOW IF I HAVE IT?

Your doctor will use a special x-ray known as a CT or MRI to figure out whether you have a brain tumor. If one is found, you will also likely have a CT/MRI or other tests on the rest of your body to make sure that your brain is the only place you have a tumor.

VITAMIN DEFICIENCIES

What they are

Vitamins are very important to keeping us healthy. When you don't get enough of a certain vitamin, you have what is known as a "vitamin deficiency." Vitamin deficiencies can cause many health problems, including tremors. If you have low levels of vitamin B12, you may get tremors[29] that affect both sides of your body and cause shaking in both your arms and your legs.[30] Interestingly, researchers have found that people with Parkinson's disease and multiple sclerosis often have vitamin D deficiency. It is unclear whether low vitamin D levels cause these diseases or is a result of having these diseases.[31,32]

How common are they?

Vitamin deficiencies are extremely common. Studies have shown that vitamin D levels are too low in 25 to 45 percent of people, even in sunny countries like Brazil.[33]

At what age do most people get them?

Vitamin deficiencies are most common in children and the elderly. However, you can get one at any age, particularly if you do not eat a balanced diet on a regular basis.[34]

What causes them?

Usually vitamin deficiencies are caused by not getting enough vitamins in your diet. This is often the case with B12 deficiency, although drinking too much alcohol can also lower your B12 levels. Vitamin D deficiency can be caused by not getting enough sunlight.

Is there a cure?

Yes. If you replace your missing vitamins through diet, pills, or injections, you can often treat the symptoms vitamin deficiencies are causing. It is important to fix any vitamin deficiency under the supervision of your doctor, because sometimes having too much of a particular vitamin in your body can cause problems, too. If your vitamin deficiency has been going on for many years, you could possibly have permanent damage to your nervous system. In those cases, your tremor may not get better even when your vitamin levels are back to normal.

How do I know if I have them?

Your doctor will run a blood test to find out if you have low levels of vitamins. You will usually have other blood levels tested at the same time as vitamins, to see if you have any problems that could be caused by vitamin deficiencies.

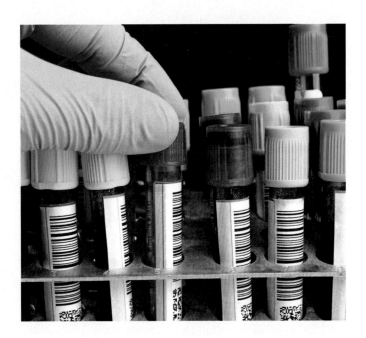

SUMMARY: WHY AM I SHAKING?

Below is a table that highlights the important features of tremor caused by the various conditions described in the last three chapters. These are general guidelines, and there are always exceptions. Do not attempt to diagnosis yourself using this chart or anything else you read in this book. Please see your doctor for a full evaluation of your tremor.

Condition	Age	When do you shake?		Where did your shaking start?		Other problems
		At rest	During an action	One side	Both sides	
"Natural" tremor	ANY	X	X		X	None
Essential tremor	ANY		X		X	None
Parkinson's disease	50s-60s 30s-40s	X		X		Stiffness Slowness Balance trouble
Hyperthyroidism	ANY		X		X	Racing heart Weight loss
Multiple sclerosis	20-40		X	X	X	Weakness Stiffness Vision trouble
Stroke	>55	X	X	X		Weakness *FAST
Brain tumor	ANY	X	X	X		Weakness Seizures Headaches
Vitamin deficiency	ANY <16 >70	X	X		X	Pain Tiredness Getting sick often

Darlene A Mayo MD FAANS   **STOP SPILLING YOUR SOUP!   The Complete Essential Tremor Solution**

REFERENCES

1. Elias WJ, Shah BB. Tremor. *JAMA.* 2014;311(9):948-954.

2. Thenganatt MA, Louis ED. Distinguishing essential tremor from Parkinson's disease: bedside tests and laboratory evaluations. *Expert Rev Neurother.* 2012;12(6):687-696.

3. Baumann CR. Epidemiology, diagnosis and differential diagnosis in Parkinson's disease tremor. *Parkinsonism Relat Disord.* 2012;18(Suppl 1):S90-2.

4. Louis ED, Clark LN, Ottman R. Familial aggregation and co-aggregation of essential tremor and Parkinson's disease. *Neuroepidemiology.* 2016;46(1):31-36.

5. The Michael J. Fox Foundation. Parkinson's diagnosis questions. https://www.michaeljfox.org/understanding-parkinsons/i-have-got-what.php.

6. Deng H, Wang P, Jankovic J. The genetics of Parkinson disease. *Ageing Res Rev.* 2017;42:72-85.

7. Borghammer P. Perfusion and metabolism imaging studies in Parkinson's disease. *Dan Med J.* 2012;59(6):B4466.

8. Milanov I, Sheinkova G. Clinical and electromyographic examination of tremor in patients with thyrotoxicosis. *Int J Clin Pract.* 2000;54(6):364-7.

9. Drugs.com. Synthroid Side Effects. https://www.drugs.com/sfx/synthroid-side-effects.html.

10. De Leo S, Lee SY, Braverman LE. Hyperthyroidism. *Lancet.* 2016;388(10047):906-918.

11. Wood-Allum CA, Shaw PJ. Thyroid disease and the nervous system. *Handb Clin Neurol.* 2014;120:703-35.

12. Fox RJ, Bacon TE, Chamot E, et al. Prevalence of multiple sclerosis symptoms across lifespan: data from the NARCOMS Registry. *Neurodegener Dis Manag.* 2015;5(6s):3-10.

13. Bötzel K, Tronnier V, Gasser T. The differential diagnosis and treatment of tremor. *Dtsch Arztebl Int.* 2014;111(13):225-236.

14. Mayr WT, Pittock SJ, McClelland RL, Jorgensen NW, Noseworthy JH, Rodriguez M. Incidence and prevalence of multiple sclerosis in Olmsted County, Minnesota, 1985-2000. *Neurology.* 2003;61(10):1373-7.

15. Ascherio A, Munger KL. Epidemiology of multiple sclerosis: environmental factors. In: Lucchinetti CF, Hohlfeld R, eds. *Multiple Sclerosis 3: Blue Books of Neurology Series, Volume 34.* Philadelphia, PA: Saunders; 2010: 58-60.

16. Garg N, Smith TW. An update on immunopathogenesis, diagnosis, and treatment of multiple sclerosis. *Brain Behav.* 2015;5(9):e00362.

17. Skovgaard L , Nicolajscn PH, Pedersen E, et al. Use of complementary and alternative medicine among people with multiple sclerosis in the Nordic countries. *Autoimmune Dis.* 2012;2012:841085.

18. National Stroke Association. Act FAST. http://www.stroke.org/understand-stroke/recognizing-stroke/act-fast.

19. Benjamin EJ, Blaha MJ, Chiuve SE, et al. Heart disease and stroke statistics—2017 update: a report from the American Heart Association. *Circulation.* 2017;135(10):e146-e603.

20. Chung LS, Tkach A, Lingenfelter EM, et al. tPA prescription and administration errors within a regional stroke system. *J Stroke Cerebrovasc Dis*. 2016;25(3):565-571.

21. Simon A, Langan A, Cooke J. Increasing efficacy of thrombectomy by using digital subtraction angiography to confirm stent retriever clot integration. *Cureus*. 2016;8(4):e559.

22. Schiff D, Lee EQ, Nayak L, Norden AD, Reardon DA, Wen PY. Medical management of brain tumors and the sequelae of treatment. *Neuro Oncol*. 2015;17(4):488-504.

23. Forsyth PA, Posner JB. Headaches in patients with brain tumors: a study of 111 patients. *Neurology*. 1993;43(9):1678-83.

24. Kurth T, Buring JR, Rist PM. Headache, migraine and risk of brain tumors in women: prospective cohort study. *J Headache Pain*. 2015;16(1):17.

25. Crawford P, Zimmerman EE. Differentiation and diagnosis of tremor. *Am Fam Physician*. 2011;83(6):697-702.

26. Bondy ML, Scheurer ME, Malmer B, et al. Brain tumor epidemiology: consensus from the Brain Tumor Epidemiology Consortium. Cancer. 2008;113(7 Suppl):1953–1968.

27. Ostrom QT, Bauchet L, Davis FG, et al. The epidemiology of glioma in adults: a "state of the science" review. *Neuro-Oncology*. 2014;16(7)896-913.

28. Hess CW, Pullman SL. Tremor: clinical phenomenology and assessment techniques. *Tremor Other Hyperkinet Mov (N Y)*. 2012;2:tre-02-65-365-1.

29. de Souza A, Moloi MW. Involuntary movements due to vitamin B12 deficiency. *Neurol Res*. 2014;36(12):1121-8.

30. Koussa S, Taher A, Sayegh R. [Postural and kinetic tremor associated with vitamin B12 deficiency]. *Rev Neurol (Paris)*. 2003;159(12):1173-4. [in French]

31. Mpandzou G, Aït Ben Haddou E, Regragui W, Benomar A, Yahyaoui M. Vitamin D deficiency and its role in neurological conditions: a review. *Rev Neurol (Paris)*. 2016;172(2):109-22.

32. Chitsaz A, Maracy M, Basiri K, et al. 25-hydroxyvitamin D and severity of Parkinson's disease. *Int J Endocrinol*. 2013;2013:689149.

33. Pereira-Santos M, Santos JYGD, Carvalho GQ, Santos DBD, Oliveira AM. Epidemiology of vitamin D insufficiency and deficiency in a population in a sunny country: geospatial meta-analysis in Brazil. *Crit Rev Food Sci Nutr*. Feb 2018:0. doi: 10.1080/10408398.2018.1437711.

34. Mithal A, Wahl DA, Bonjour JP, et al. Global vitamin D status and determinants of hypovitaminosis D. *Osteoporos Int*. 2009;20:1807-1820.

RELATED PROBLEMS

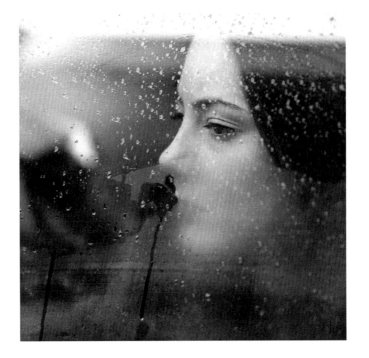

It is very common for people who have tremors to also have other problems, such as depression and anxiety.[1] On one level, this makes all the sense in the world. When you shake and cannot do the things that you need or want to do, it can make you feel sad. Also, it can be embarrassing to go out in public when you shake.

People who do not understand that tremors are often caused by medical conditions or diseases can sometimes seem to be judging you. Patients have told me that they have been asked if they were "coming off a bender" when people have seen them shaking in a store. Sometimes, you may feel that others are giving you judgmental looks when you try to eat in a restaurant. This can make you not want to go out in public, and if you do go out, you may feel very anxious. As mentioned in the first chapter of this book, anxiety can make your tremors worse.

What you also may not realize is that there are changes in the brains of people with tremors that are connected to anxiety and depression. It is unclear whether the brain changes that cause essential tremor (ET) and Parkinson's disease (PD) also cause anxiety and depression, or if the anxiety and depression you feel because of experiences with tremor lead to those brain changes.[2,3]

DEPRESSION

Depression is a psychological term to describe sadness or a feeling of hopelessness that lasts two weeks or longer.[4] If you were, for example, going through a period of grief after a loved one has died, then this sadness would generally **not** be considered depression. However, if you feel continued sadness due to a chronic (long-term) medical condition such as ET, or a disease such as PD, this would qualify. Depression is also more than just sadness. It can make you feel a lack of energy or motivation to do anything and a lack of interest in activities that used to bring you pleasure, such as hobbies. Severe depression could make you not even want to get out bed, or could possibly make you feel suicidal. If you think that you may be depressed, I urge you to seek medical treatment immediately.

Certainly, if you have any thoughts about hurting yourself, please call the following number and talk to someone right now, or go to your local emergency room.

1-800-SUICIDE (784-2433)[5]

Know that you are not alone. Between 25 and 60 percent of people with ET and up to 70 percent of people with PD develop depression at some point during their lifetime.[3,6]

There are a number of medicines, counseling options, and other treatments that can be very helpful for depression. If you think you are or are becoming depressed, please contact your doctor as soon as possible. With treatment, depression can get better.[4]

Anxiety is a condition that can be described as severe nervousness or worry that lasts for a few months or more.[7] Anxiety affects about 33 to 42 percent of people with ET and around 60 to 70 percent of people with PD.[3,6] Severe anxiety can also lead to panic attacks or a condition called "social phobia." During a panic attack, you may think you are having a heart attack. Your heart races, you may feel like you cannot breathe, or you may start breathing very fast. Panic attacks can come on at any time. They are often caused by a moment of fear and usually only last for a few moments. The deep breathing and meditation techniques described in Section 2 can help make panic attacks shorter and less intense. You may have social phobia if you are fearful of going out in public places. About 14 percent of people with ET experience this.[2] Anxiety in general and social phobia in particular can make you want to avoid going out to eat or having any social interactions at all.

As with depression, there are a number of medicines and counseling techniques that can help you overcome or at least lessen your anxiety.[7] If you think you have anxiety, I urge you to talk to your doctor immediately. Treatment of anxiety can help you not only feel less anxious, but also decrease your tremor.[1]

REFERENCES

1. Achey RL, Yamamoto E, Sexton D, et al. Prediction of depression and anxiety via patient-assessed tremor severity, not physician-reported motor symptom severity, in patients with Parkinson's disease or essential tremor who have undergone deep brain stimulation. *J Neurosurg.* 2018;23:1-10.

2. Louis ED. Non-motor symptoms in essential tremor: a review of the current data and state of the field. *Parkinsonism Relat Disord.* 2016;22(Suppl 1):S115-S118.

3. Kulisevsky J, Pagonabarraga J, Pascual-Sedano B, García-Sánchez C, Gironell A. Prevalence and correlates of neuropsychiatric symptoms in Parkinson's disease without dementia. *Mov Disord.* 2008;23(13):1889-96.

4. National Institute of Mental Health. Depression. http://www.nimh.nih.gov/health/topics/depression/index.shtml. Revised February 2018.

5. MentalHealth.net. Depression Hotline Number. http://www.mentalhelp.net/articles/depression-hotline. Published May 30, 2017. Updated June 20, 2017.

6. Smeltere L, Kuzņecovs V, Erts R. Depression and social phobia in essential tremor and Parkinson's disease. *Brain Behav.* 2017;7(9):e00781.

7. National Institute of Mental Health. Anxiety Disorders. http://www.nimh.nih.gov/health/topics/anxiety-disorders/index.shtml. Revised March 2016.

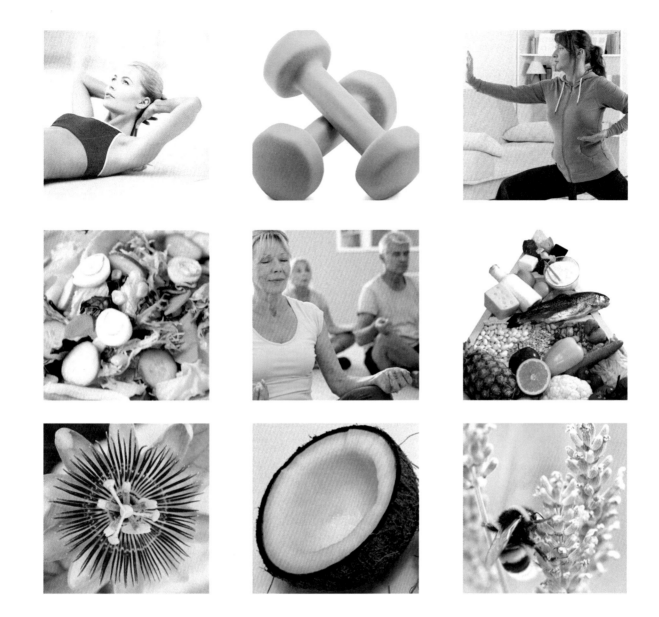

SECTION

2

AT HOME TREATMENTS

ACTIVITIES THAT SLOW DOWN TREMORS

I have noticed that when my patients first come to see me, and when I lead essential tremor (ET) support groups, most people believe nothing can be done for tremors outside of taking medicine or possibly having surgery. This is simply not true! There are a number of ways that you, yourself, can help decrease your tremors, and not one of these requires that you set foot in a doctor's office.

In a recent survey of over 1400 people with ET, a large percentage of people said that they wanted a "wider range" of treatment choices for ET beyond medicine and surgery. In particular, many said they would like to see more options like exercises and alternative treatments to help them do their day-to-day activities.[1]

In this chapter, I will describe a few activities, such as easy at-home exercises, tai chi, yoga, meditation, and visualization techniques, that can help you control your tremor starting today.

EASY EXERCISES TO STRENGTHEN YOUR MUSCLES

Strengthening the muscles of your arms and midsection, or "core," is a great way to decrease your tremor. Muscles that are weak have to work much harder to do anything. So, weak muscles can actually bring out "natural" tremor in almost anyone, particularly if you already have a medical condition that causes you to shake. By strengthening these muscles through daily exercise, your arms will not have to work as hard to turn a door knob or hold a coffee cup. A little bit goes a long way—you do not have to power lift weights at a gym to see results. These simple exercises done consistently, daily or every other day, will strengthen most people's muscles in a few weeks.

> BY STRENGTHENING MUSCLES THROUGH DAILY EXERCISE, YOUR ARMS WILL NOT HAVE TO WORK AS HARD TO TURN A DOOR KNOB OR HOLD A COFFEE CUP.

WHAT RESULTS CAN I EXPECT?

Research in this area is just beginning. There are very few studies that have looked at the impact of specific exercises on tremor. The research that has been done suggests that physical activity and resistance (strength) training can reduce tremors caused by ET and Parkinson's disease (PD).[2-6] It takes some time to build up muscle strength, so expect it to take a few months of exercise before you start to see improvement in your tremors.

WHAT EXERCISES SHOULD I DO?

The exercises described below are general exercises to increase your muscle strength. They are adapted from different websites.[7-10] They should be fairly easy for you if you are in good overall health. I recommend that you talk to your doctor before trying this or any other exercise program. Also, if you see an occupational therapist (a person who can help you manage your tremor in your daily life), he or she may slightly change these exercises or give you different exercises to try. See Section 3 of this book for more information about how an occupational therapist can help you.

I also encourage you to do some gentle stretches before and after you exercise. This is very important, as it decreases the chance you will injure your muscles. Stretches can be as simple as making big circles with your arms a few times and opening your hands as widely as you can and closing them a few times.

For some of these exercises, I have recommended certain amounts of weight you can use. These are ranges only. The goal is for you to find the weight that, after 8 to 10 repetitions (numbers of times you do a specific exercise), makes your muscles feel almost too tired to do one more repetition. You may need to test out different weights for the first couple of days you do these exercises. You can usually buy weights to use at home from any big-box store (such as Walmart or Target). Also, keep in mind that you may not be ready for weights, particularly if you have not exercised in a while. It is just fine (and still helpful!) to do these exercises without any weights until your muscles start to get stronger. If you exercise without weights, concentrate on tightening your muscles when you do each exercise. This will help make your muscles stronger.

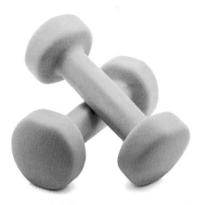

ARM, WRIST, AND HAND EXERCISES

Arm curls

Weight: 3 lbs. to 5 lbs.

Technique: Sit down in a chair or on a bench. Keep your elbow close to your side, near the bottom of your rib cage. Keep your palm up, facing the ceiling. If you are using a weight, then put it in your hand after you are in this position. Bend your elbow and raise your arm until it touches your shoulder. Then, slowly lower your arm back down. Do 8 to 10 repetitions on one side, then switch the weight to your other hand and repeat. You should feel a stretch in your bicep, which is the muscle in the front of your upper arm.

> **IMPORTANT NOTES:**
>
> 1. As with all exercise, if you feel any pain and are doing this without a trained professional watching you, you must stop exercising immediately!
>
> 2. If you decide to use weights with any of these exercises, please be careful! If your tremor is so severe that you drop things often, then please pay attention to where the weight will fall if you drop it, and do not use weights for any exercises that involve lifting your arms above your head.

Wrist curls forward

Weight: 1 lb. to 3 lbs.

Technique: You can do this either sitting or standing. Extend one arm straight out from your body, so that it is parallel with the floor. Keep your palm down, facing the floor. If you are using a weight, be sure you stay in this position while the weight is in your hand. Bend your wrist down slowly, and then bend it back up. Be careful not to let gravity do the work for you. Do 8 to 10 repetitions on one side, then switch the weight to the other side and repeat. You should feel a stretch in the back of your lower arm, between your elbow and wrist.

> NOTE: If this is too hard for you to do with your arm unsupported, then sit in a chair that has arm rests. Rest your forearm on the arm rest, so that your wrist extends just over the front edge of the arm rest. Then, continue with the exercise as described above. Once you gain enough strength, you can do the exercise without your arm supported.

Wrist curls reversed

Weight: 1 lb. to 3 lbs.

Technique: You can do this either sitting or standing. Extend one arm straight out from your body, so that it is parallel with the floor. Keep your palm up, facing the ceiling. If you are using a weight, be sure you stay in this position while the weight is in your hand. Bend your wrist down slowly, and then bend it back up. Be careful not to let gravity do the work for you. Do 8 to 10 repetitions on one side, then switch the weight to the other side and repeat. You should feel a stretch in the front of your lower arm, between your elbow and the wrist.

> NOTE: If this is too hard for you to do with your arm unsupported, then sit in a chair that has arm rests. Rest your forearm on the arm rest, so that your wrist extends just over the front edge of the arm rest. Then, continue with the exercise as described above. Once you gain enough strength, you can do the exercise without your arm supported.

Finger strengthening

Weight: none

Equipment: Stress ball

Technique: Sit down in a chair or on a bench. Rest your arms on your lap. Hold the stress ball in one hand and squeeze it tightly for 10 seconds. Release the ball. Rest for 5 seconds. Repeat 8 to 10 times with each hand. You will feel a stretch in your fingers.

CORE EXERCISES

You may think that strengthening the muscles in your hands and arms is enough. While this can help decrease the chance that you will shake when you are holding a cup or utensil, what can help even more are exercises to make your "core" (midsection) stronger. The reason these exercises help is that your core will support your movement more so that your arms and legs do not have to do as much "work." The less work your arms have to do, the less likely you are to shake. You do not have to get a "body-builder" physique to make a difference!

Below are a few exercises that will help you get a stronger core. If you have not exercised in a while, please talk to your doctor before starting any of these. And as with the exercises above, if you feel any pain, stop immediately. You can do these exercises every day, or you can do them 2 or 3 times a week—anything should help! The exercises are listed in order from easy to hard.

CORE MUSCLE CONTRACTIONS

Weight: none

Technique: You can do this while standing or sitting. Be sure your back is straight and your shoulders are pulled back. Tighten your stomach muscles and hold for 10 seconds. Remember to breathe while your muscles are tightened! Release your muscles. Rest for 5 seconds. Repeat 8 to 10 times. You will feel a stretch in your midsection and possibly your back.

SIDE STRETCHES

Weight: 1 lb. to 3 lbs. if desired

Technique: While sitting in a chair, plant your feet firmly on the ground. Rest your left hand in your lap. Raise your right arm above your head and place it next to your ear. Now, bend your upper body at your waist to the left. This is not a rotation. You should feel a stretch along the side of your body. Now bring your body back upright. Repeat this 8 to 10 times. Then, switch arms, and repeat the exercise on the other side of your body.

CRUNCHES

Equipment: none

Technique: Lie down on the floor with your back flat, knees bent, and feet flat on the floor. Place your hands behind your head. Contract your abdominal muscles and raise your head and shoulders a few inches off the ground, toward your knees. Try not to pull your head up using your arms. If you can only raise your head and shoulders slightly off the ground, that is fine. Stay in this position for 5 seconds. Then, slowly lower your head and upper body back down to the ground. Repeat 8 to 10 times. You can increase the number of repetitions you do as you get stronger. You will feel a stretch in your midsection and possibly your lower back.

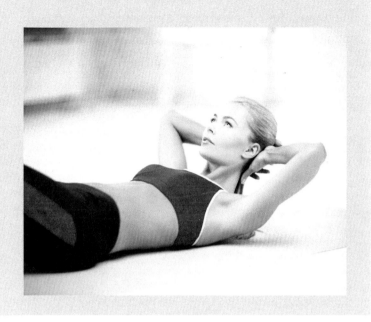

TAI CHI TO "RETRAIN YOUR BRAIN"

What it is and how it works

Tai chi is a type of Chinese martial art that focuses on smooth, flowing body movements. It involves very gentle stretches done in a standing position. It is technically a type of exercise; however, it is very easy on your body and joints. Almost anyone can do the moves in tai chi. It can help decrease stress, improve balance, and increase flexibility. It is not well understood how tai chi helps lessen tremors, but you can think of it like this. By practicing smooth, flowing movements, these patterns, or pathways, in your brain will get reinforced instead of the "tremor pathways." In this way, tai chi can "retrain your brain" to make smoother movements.

Where to find tai chi classes

You can often find tai chi classes at community centers, your local YMCA, colleges, gyms, or karate training centers. Some centers that offer yoga may also offer tai chi classes. You should look for beginner tai chi classes, as there are other types of tai chi that may be too challenging for you initially.

What to expect during the class

Most tai chi classes last about 60 minutes. You should wear loose-fitting clothes to help with the flow of the movements. You will start with some gentle stretching and breathing techniques. Then, your instructor will guide you into the flowing movements. Many of the movements are repetitive. The repetition of physical activity is great for strengthening brain pathways, such as those that make smooth movements.[11,12] It is also helpful if you spend a few minutes every day between formal classes doing some of the tai chi movements you have learned.

What results can I expect?

Tai chi has been shown to improve movement, balance, and walking in people with PD.[13] It can also help people think through problems more clearly.[14] Many anecdotal (individual) reports have shown tai chi reduced or "cured" tremors in people with PD and ET; however, researchers have not yet formally studied this. Because tai chi has no known side effects, if you do it in a class setting with a qualified instructor, it may a safe option for you to help improve your tremors.

How much does it cost?

Most tai chi classes cost about $15 to $20. Some centers offer monthly packages that further lower that cost. Most insurance companies will not cover tai chi classes. There is a bill currently being considered in Congress called the Personal Health Investment Today (PHIT) Act. If passed, this bill will allow the cost of certain exercise classes, equipment, and gym memberships to be deducted from your taxes (up to $1000 per year).[15] Tai chi classes would be covered by this bill.

YOGA SESSIONS TO STRENGTHEN AND RELAX YOU

WHAT IT IS AND HOW IT WORKS

Yoga is a combination of practices, including stretching and strength exercises, breathing techniques, and meditation. There are many types of yoga. Some focus on holding poses for long or short periods of time in order to build strength, while others focus more on flowing movement, similar to what you would find in a tai chi class. Some classes combine these two techniques or offer other types of yoga as well. Yoga likely helps decrease tremors by activating the parasympathetic nervous system (see Section 4) and by strengthening the muscles. The repetitive poses also likely help build and reinforce brain pathways of smooth movement, as described in the tai chi section above.

WHERE TO FIND YOGA CLASSES

You can find yoga classes in many of the same places you will find tai chi classes. There are also yoga studios that offer many types of yoga classes, from beginner to expert levels. Classes may also be offered at some gyms, the YMCA, or your local community center or college. Some places of business now offer yoga classes early in the morning, around lunch breaks, or after work to give employees a chance to relax during the workday. Certification is not required for yoga instructors; however, you may want to search on the Yoga Alliance website (https://www.yogaalliance.org) to find a certified yoga instructor. This certification ensures that instructors have a minimum level of training that can help class participants avoid injury.

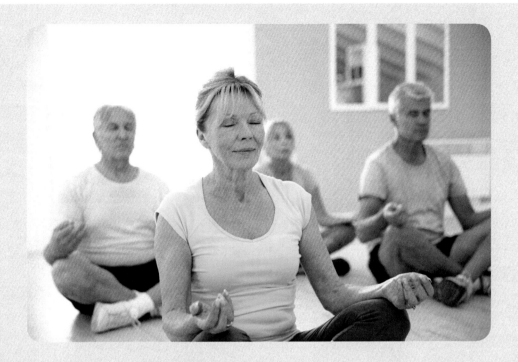

WHAT TO EXPECT DURING THE CLASS

Most yoga classes last 60-90 minutes, depending on the type of yoga and whether you are taking a beginner-, advanced-, or expert-level class. Dress comfortably in clothes that stretch easily. If you have long hair, you will want to tie it up to keep it out of your face during some of the poses. Generally, your instructor will start by introducing himself or herself and ask if anyone is new to yoga or has any limitations. Either at this point, or before the class if you feel more comfortable, you may want to mention that you have tremors. The instructor may suggest changes you can make to certain poses to make them easier for you to manage.

Most instructors will begin with some breathing exercises. After this, you will do some easier poses and then progress to more challenging ones. At any point during a yoga class, if you feel that something is too difficult, you can move into one of a few "resting poses" that your instructor will teach you in the beginning of class. Once you feel stronger, you can return to the poses that the rest of the class is doing. There are also "chair yoga" classes that may be easier for you if you are just getting started.

WHAT RESULTS CAN I EXPECT?

One study has looked into whether yoga can reduce shaking. In this study,[16] people attended yoga sessions two to three times per week for several weeks. Researchers found that tremors decreased in people with PD for several hours after each yoga session. There was no long-term follow up to see if the sessions had any lasting effects on tremor. No studies have been done to explore the effects of yoga on tremors from ET, but there are several anecdotal reports that yoga can improve these tremors. As with tai chi, participating in a yoga class with a qualified instructor guiding you has a very low risk of injury.

HOW MUCH DOES IT COST?

Most yoga classes cost about $10 to $20. Some centers may offer monthly packages that further lower that cost. Occasionally, some places offer free yoga classes. These classes often request a donation of $5 to $10. Most insurance companies will not cover yoga. If passed, the PHIT Act[15] described above would allow you to deduct the cost of yoga classes from your taxes as a medical expense.

MEDITATION TO RELAX YOUR MIND AND YOUR BODY

What it is and how it works

Meditation is a practice that helps you rest and clear your mind and relax your body.

When you learn to do this, you will often start by focusing your mind on one single thought for a period of time. By focusing on one thing, you will become better able to "empty your mind" of all the thoughts that have been worrying you. The art of meditation has been practiced for thousands of years. Sometimes the idea of meditation may seem a little "out there" for some people. But when you look at the vast amount of research that has been done on the benefits of meditation,[17-21] you may find it very hard to remain skeptical.

One thing I love about meditation is that there is science behind it. I do not think we fully understand this, but scientific research shows that meditation changes the way your brain cells "talk" to one another.[22,23] Brain cells in people with tremor often have trouble "talking" to one another normally, so it makes sense that meditation could be helpful.

What results can I expect?

As mentioned above, there are many scientific studies that show ways in which meditation can improve your health, including helping you lose weight, making you less depressed and anxious, and improving your ability to think through problems.[17-21] Interestingly, meditation's ability to control tremor has not been formally studied. There is a single case study that describes a person whose tremors due to PD were "cured" with regular meditation practice.[24] There are also many anecdotal reports that meditation can improve tremors even after a single meditation session.[17] To see the most improvement in your tremors, though, you will need to meditate regularly over a period of many weeks or months.

How can I meditate when I am anxious?

Having anxiety can make it challenging to feel like you will get anywhere when you first start meditating. Believe me, I understand what you are feeling. You think you will not be able to focus on one thing for five seconds, much less five minutes. Let me tell you that you **can** learn to do this—I did! As a neurosurgeon with people's lives in my hands every day, I had every reason to feel stressed. I had hundreds of anxious thoughts running through my mind every day. I found it very difficult to relax and stay focused on a single thought for even a minute when I first started meditating. Now, after a few years of regular practice, I can meditate for almost an hour at a time.

Meditation takes time and practice (as do most things). But it is by far one of the most rewarding things I have ever learned to do. Not only does meditation help me with stress, but it helps me with almost everything in my life—from writing this book and running my business to parenting my children.

So how do I start meditating?

- *You start small and work your way up.*
- *You give yourself grace and patience.*
- *You treat yourself kindly as you are learning.*

Below I will explain a simple meditation method I use that works well for me. Try this. Try it for five minutes. If that seems too long, try it for two minutes, or even one minute. Then try it again tomorrow. Keep working on it each day for a few days. It will get easier. On some days it might be easier to meditate than on others. That is completely normal. If you are not "feeling it" one day, then skip that day and try again the next day.

If you try this meditation technique, and you just do not feel like it "fits" you, there are hundreds of other techniques you can use. On my website (www.helpfortremors.com), I have a blog post that lists meditation resources that have been helpful to me.

Darlene A Mayo MD FAANS   **STOP SPILLING YOUR SOUP!**   The Complete Essential Tremor Solution

A focused meditation technique

The first time you do this, I recommend you set a timer for five minutes. See how you feel at the end of your meditation time. If you feel like you could have meditated longer, try adding more time the next day. If five minutes seemed like an eternity, shorten it to three minutes the next day and work your way up to longer meditation times.

NOTE: The timer alarm you set should ideally be something gentle and peaceful. If you use a cell phone, set a nice tone or melody that will help ease you out of your meditation.

LOCATION AND POSTURE

- *Go to a quiet place in your house or outdoors.*
- *Sit upright with your back straight or lie down. (Try not to fall asleep!)*
- *Turn your palms down on the arms of a chair, on the ground, or in your lap. You can also place your hands together in a traditional prayer position if you prefer.*
- *Close your eyes if you feel comfortable doing so.*

BREATHING

- *Take a deep breath in through your nose or mouth. Count slowly to five while you do this. Then breathe out just as slowly, again counting to five.*
- *As you breathe in deeply, see if you can make not only your chest but also your belly rise. Then, when you are breathing out, feel your belly go down and your chest pull in.*
- *Take three breaths like this. How do you feel? Are you starting to feel calmer? Sometimes it is helpful to repeat this for another three breaths—or more—on days when it is hard to calm down.*
- *Now, breathe normally.*

FOCUS

- *Choose a word you want to focus on. Make it something positive and calming, like "peace," "calm," or "hope." It does not really matter what the word is, as long as you associate the word with something pleasant.*
- *Each time you take a breath in, say your word silently in your head.*
- *When you breathe out, let your mind go blank. This gives your brain time to relax.*

NOTE: Thoughts may come into your head while you do this. This is okay and totally normal. The idea of meditation is not to do it "perfectly" but to keep practicing until it gets easier. Meditating, or learning to "calm your brain," is an "exercise" for your brain. Just as you cannot expect to start lifting 50-pound weights right away without practice, you cannot expect to keep a completely clear mind while meditating without practice.

ENDING YOUR MEDITATION TIME

- *When your timer goes off, wait a moment before opening your eyes.*
- *Wiggle your fingers and toes a bit, then slowly open your eyes.*
- *Breathe deeply for a couple of minutes, then ease yourself back into your day.*

Once you start meditating daily, you will find yourself feeling calmer. As you learn to calm your brain, your tremor will also slow down.

What it is and how it works

Along with meditation, another powerful technique to help control your tremor is visualization. Visualization simply means imagining something and creating an image of it in your mind. Visualization, particularly when used in combination with meditation, can be a very powerful way to create realistic pictures in your mind. This concept, also called "mental imagery," can help people improve their physical performance. Studies have shown that athletes who spend time imagining all the details of their performance, over and over, actually perform better than those who spend that same amount of time only training their bodies.[25,26]

It may seem rather amazing that this can actually work. Did you know that it is very hard for your brain to tell the difference between an imagined movement and a real movement? The same brain cells are activated in both cases! These brain cells are called "mirror neurons," because they react in a similar way to both real and imagined movements.[27,28] So, when you visualize your arm moving, you can make your brain "think" your arm is actually moving. This is how visualization can help athletes perform better and how it can also help control your tremor.

What results can I expect?

Research on the power of visualization is quite strong. In addition to helping athletes perform, visualization helps people recover from injuries such as stroke faster than people who only have standard physical therapy.[28,29] You may wonder if the power of visualization will work as well if you have a chronic condition that affects your brain (like ET or PD). A few years ago, researchers thought this might be a problem.[30] However, in two recent studies, the brains of an ET patient and several patients with PD showed strong, regular signals when the patients imagined moving their hands.[31,32] This has led other researchers to believe that visualization may help improve symptoms such as tremor in patients with ET and Parkinson's disease.[33]

How do I start visualizing?

To reduce your tremors, you will imagine yourself doing the things you love to do but without shaking. This may seem impossible, but it is not. I will guide you through a way to do this that will work for anyone—whether or not you think you have a good imagination.

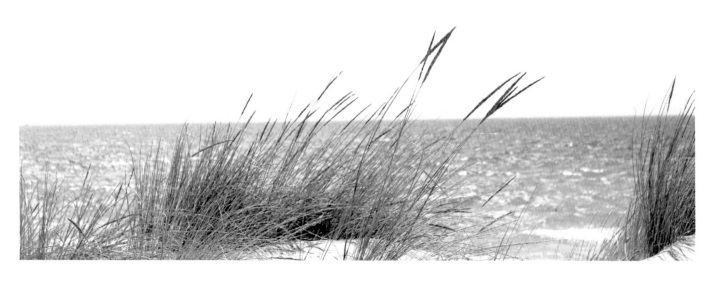

PREPARE FOR YOUR VISUALIZATION

The first thing you should do is decide what you want to imagine. What would you most love to do but have trouble doing because of your tremor? Would you like to drink water without spilling it? Get your key in your front door on the first try? Or maybe your greatest desire is to be able to play golf, or crochet again. Whatever it is, decide now.

I will wait.

Now that you have decided what is most important to you, think about every detail of this experience. For example, if you chose "eat soup without spilling it," you would think about the following:

- What kind of soup do you want to eat? Chicken noodle? Split pea? Tomato?
- In what kind of bowl do you want to eat it? China? Plastic?
- Where do you want to eat your soup? At a dining room table? In your favorite restaurant?
- With whom do you want to share the experience? Your family? A special friend?
- How will you feel when you can eat a whole bowl of soup without spilling it?

Now, your next step is to either write down all of these details or, if your tremor makes it hard for you to write, say them out loud. If you choose to say them out loud, record yourself or have someone else record you so that you can play it back later.

As you write or speak, create in your mind a very detailed image of each of these items.

START VISUALIZING

Now, you are going to visualize yourself actually eating the soup. You will imagine the whole process, from sitting down at the table, to picking up the spoon, to putting the first spoonful in your mouth. Once you swallow the soup, you will get another spoonful.

As you start to visualize, add in other details. How does the spoon feel in your hand? Is it heavy? Is the soup hot or warm? What does it smell like? What does it taste like as you are eating it? What sounds do you hear? Are you so hungry or maybe so excited to be eating soup that you gulp it down? How satisfied do you feel after you have eaten the first spoonful?

Now, repeat this whole process, making one important change: **Imagine yourself doing all of these things—without any shaking in your hand.**

See yourself picking up the spoon smoothly and with ease. See yourself holding it in your hand for a minute. Watch in wonder at how steady it is! Now, put the spoon in the bowl of soup. Do it smoothly, not hitting the sides of the bowl, and get a full spoonful of soup. Now see yourself bringing the spoon to your mouth. Not one drop will fall off the spoon. Now put the spoon in your mouth. How amazing does that taste?

That is all there is to it! Repeat this process of visualization a few times a day. Stick with the same visualization for a while before trying to imagine other things (e.g., turning a key in a lock, writing clearly, etc.).

First, just like with meditation, the more you practice visualization, the easier it will become. The images will become more vivid, and you will be better able to use your five senses (seeing, smelling, tasting, touch, and hearing) in your visualization.

Second, the more often you use visualization, the better your results will be.

Lastly, for some people it is easier to do visualization while they are meditating. So, for example, after you have done the breathing part of your meditation (see section above) and repeated your chosen word a couple of times, you could start your visualization.

Try visualization, and see how your tremor is day by day, week by week. You may start to notice that your tremor is just a little better than it was, or that there are longer periods of time during which your tremor is under control. The power of the mind is amazing. Try this and see what it can do.

REFERENCES

1. Louis ED, Rohl B, Rice C. Defining the treatment gap: what essential tremor patients want that they are not getting. *Tremor Other Hyperkinet Mov (N Y)*. 2015;5:331.

2. Louis ED, Collins K, Rohl B, et al. Self-reported physical activity in essential tremor: relationship with tremor, balance, and cognitive function. *J Neurol Sci*. 2016;366:240-245.

3. Kavanagh JJ, Wedderburn-Bisshop J, Keogh JW. Resistance training reduces force tremor and improves manual dexterity in older individuals with essential tremor. *J Mot Behav*. 2016;48(1):20-30.

4. Bilodeau M, Keen DA, Sweeney PJ, Shields RW, Enoka RM. Strength training can improve steadiness in persons with essential tremor. *Muscle Nerve*. 2000;23(5):771-8.

5. Earhart GM, Falvo MJ. Parkinson disease and exercise. *Compr Physiol*. 2013;3(2):833-48.

6. Shulman LM, Katzel LI, Ivey FM, et al. Randomized clinical trial of 3 types of physical exercise for patients with Parkinson disease. *JAMA Neurology*. 2013;70(2):183–190.

7. Zehr M. How to Treat Hand Tremors by Exercising. Livestrong.com. https://www.livestrong.com/article/449077-how-to-cure-hand-tremors-by-exercising. Published September 11, 2017.

8. Harrison L. 7 Exercises to Maximize Hand, Wrist, and Forearm Strength. BreakingMuscle. https://breakingmuscle.com/fitness/7-exercises-to-maximize-hand-wrist-and-forearm-strength. Published February 2017.

9. Elkaim Y. 7 Best Abdominal Exercises for Seniors (Do These Anywhere). YuriElkaim. https://yurielkaim.com/abdominal-exercises-for-seniors.

10. wikiHow. How to Exercise Your Abs While Sitting. https://www.wikihow.fitness/Exercise-Your-Abs-While-Sitting.

11. Engeroff T, Vogt L, Fleckenstein J, et al. Lifespan leisure physical activity profile, brain plasticity and cognitive function in old age. *Aging Ment Health*. Jan 2018:1-8. doi: 10.1080/13607863.2017.1421615.

12. Tøien T, Unhjem R, Øren TS, Kvellestad ACG, Hoff J, Wang E. Neural plasticity with age: unilateral maximal strength training augments efferent neural drive to the contralateral limb in older adults. *J Gerontol A Biol Sci Med Sci*. Nov 2017. doi: 10.1093/gerona/glx218.

13. Li F, Harmer P, Fitzgerald K, et al. Tai chi and postural stability in patients with Parkinson's disease. *N Engl J Med*. 2012;366(6):511–519.

14. Yang JH, Wang YQ, Ye SQ, et al.The effects of group-based versus individual-based tai chi training on nonmotor symptoms in patients with mild to moderate Parkinson's disease: a randomized controlled pilot trial. *Parkinsons Dis*. 2017;2017:8562867.

15. United States, Congress. "Personal Health Investment Today Act or the PHIT Act." H.R. 1267, 115th Cong. 2017. https://www.congress.gov/bill/115th-congress/house-bill/1267.

16. Sharma NK, Robbins K, Wagner K, Colgrove YM. A randomized controlled pilot study of the therapeutic effects of yoga in people with Parkinson's disease. *Int J Yoga*. 2015;8(1):74-9.

17. Edwards MK, Loprinzi PD. Affective responses to acute bouts of aerobic exercise, mindfulness meditation, and combinations of exercise and meditation: a randomized controlled intervention. *Psychol Rep*. Jan 2018:33294118755099. doi: 10.1177/0033294118755099.

18. Spadaro KC, Davis KK, Sereika SM, Gibbs BB, Jakicic JM, Cohen SM. Effect of mindfulness meditation on short-term weight loss and eating behaviors in overweight and obese adults: A randomized controlled trial. *J Complement Integr Med*. Dec 2017. doi: 10.1515/jcim-2016-0048.

19. Chan RW, Immink MA, Lushington K. The influence of focused-attention meditation states on the cognitive control of sequence learning. *Conscious Cogn*. 2017;55:11-25.

20. Advocat J, Enticott J, Vandenberg B, et al. The effects of a mindfulness-based lifestyle program for adults with Parkinson's disease: a mixed methods, wait list controlled randomised control study. *BMC Neurol*. 2016;16(1):166.

21. Verma G, Araya R. The effect of meditation on psychological distress among Buddhist monks and nuns. *Int J Psychiatry Med*. 2010;40(4):461-8.

22. Chiesa A, Serretti A. A systematic review of neurobiological and clinical features of mindfulness meditations. *Psychol Med*. 2010;40(8):1239-52.

23. Marzetti L, Di Lanzo C, Zappasodi F, et al. Magnetoencephalographic alpha band connectivity reveals differential default mode network interactions during focused attention and open monitoring meditation. *Front Hum Neurosci*. 2014;8:832.

24. Smart K, Durso R, Morgan J, McNamara P. A potential case of remission of Parkinson's disease. *J Complement Integr Med*. 2016;13(3):311-315.

25. Di Rienzo F, Blache Y, Kanthack TF, Monteil K, Collet C, Guillot A. Short-term effects of integrated motor imagery practice on muscle activation and force performance. *Neuroscience*. 2015;305:146-56.

26. Battaglia C, D'Artibale E, Fiorilli G, et al. Use of video observation and motor imagery on jumping performance in national rhythmic gymnastics athletes. *Hum Mov Sci*. 2014;38:225-34.

27. di Pellegrino G, Fadiga L, Fogassi L, Gallese V, Rizzolatti G. Understanding motor events: a neurophysiological study. *Exp Brain Res*. 1992;91(1):176-80.

28. Carvalho D, Teixeira ML, Yuan TF, et al. The mirror neuron system in post-stroke rehabilitation. *Int Arch Med*. 2013;6:41.

29. Claflin ES, Krishnan C, Khot SP. Emerging treatments for motor rehabilitation after stroke. *Neurohospitalist*. 2015;5(2):77-88.

30. Lo YL, Louis ED, Fook-Chong S, Tan EK. Impaired motor imagery in patients with essential tremor: a case control study. *Mov Disord*. 2007;22(4):504-8.

31. Marquez-Chin C, Popovic MR, Sanin E, Chen R, and Lozano AM. Real-time two-dimensional asynchronous control of a computer cursor with a single subdural electrode. *J Spinal Cord Med*. 2012;35(5):382–391.

32. Helmich RC, Bloem BR, Toni I. Motor imagery evokes increased somatosensory activity in Parkinson's disease patients with tremor. *Hum Brain Mapp*. 2012;33(8):1763-79.

33. Caligiore D, Mustile M, Spalletta G, Baldassarre G. Action observation and motor imagery for rehabilitation in Parkinson's disease: a systematic review and an integrative hypothesis. *Neurosci Biobehav Rev*. 2017;72:210-222.

WHAT TO EAT AND DRINK
TO STOP SHAKING

In Section 1 of this book, I described a few of the foods and drinks that are known to make tremors due to any cause worse. In this chapter, I focus on specific changes to your diet, including food choices, herbs, and drink choices, that may decrease your tremors. Keep in mind that changes to your diet are usually most successful when you make them gradually. Also, it will often take a few weeks to see health benefits, including reduced tremor, after you make changes to your diet.

THE MEDITERRANEAN DIET

You may have heard the phrase, "You are what you eat." What this means is that the foods you eat can actually affect your body. The really good news is that eating certain types of foods can reduce your shaking! Now, I know what you're thinking: "Am I going to have to eat bean sprouts and rabbit food and be hungry all the time to stop shaking?" The answer is, "No you don't!" The diet that has been linked to reduced tremors is actually full of delicious food! And you really do not have to limit the amount of food you eat in order to reduce your tremors.

This diet is called the "Mediterranean diet," because the people who eat these foods often live near the Mediterranean Sea. Research has shown that essential tremor (ET) is far less common in people who live near the Mediterranean and eat these types of food.[1,2]

So, what foods are in the Mediterranean diet? There are many wonderful choices!

- *Fish*
- *Chicken (limited amounts)*
- *Eggs*
- *Olive oil*
- *Fresh fruits and vegetables*
- *Wheat breads and pastas*
- *Nuts*
- *Beans*
- *Red wine*

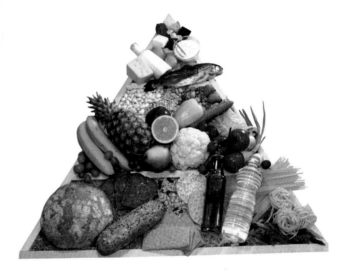

The foods you should avoid on the Mediterranean diet are foods that are not healthy for you anyway. Avoid processed foods, keep milk and cheese to a minimum, limit your meals that have red meat, and watch how much sugar is in your food. Also, it is important that you eat regularly throughout the day. For example, eating a healthy breakfast, lunch, and dinner, with a couple of small snacks in between meals, helps keep the sugar levels in your blood more even throughout the day. As mentioned in Section 1, keeping blood sugar levels regular helps keep your tremors under control.[3]

You can find a lot of information and recipe books on the Mediterranean diet that will teach you how to integrate these types of food into your life. On my website (www.helpfortremors.com), you will find links to some of the more recent books on the Mediterranean diet.

LOW MEAT/LOW HARMANE DIET

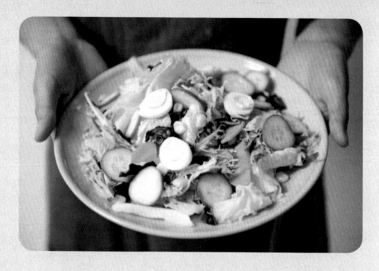

You probably know that it is healthier to eat baked rather than fried foods. You may also know that eating large amounts of meat can cause health problems. What you may not realize is that several recent studies have linked meats cooked at very high temperatures (such as during frying or grilling on an open flame) to hand tremors in general and to ET in particular.[4-6] These studies discovered that a dangerous neurotoxin (nerve poison) called "harmane" is found in high levels in the blood of people who eat a lot of meat. This is important, because people with high harmane levels are 21 times more likely to have ET! There are also many anecdotal (individual) reports that people who switched to a "plant-based," or vegetarian, diet reduced or completely stopped their tremors due to ET.

So, another way you may be able to reduce your tremors is to eat less meat, choose low-heat cooking methods (such as baking), and eat your meat less well done. Keep in mind that a blood test for harmane levels needs special laboratory equipment, so you will not be able to go to your doctor and ask to have this blood test done.

HIGH OCTANOIC ACID DIET

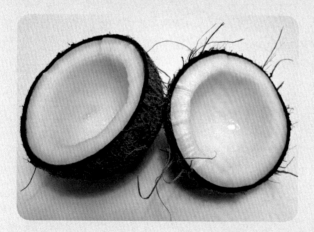

Researchers have identified a type of alcohol, called "octanoic acid," that helps decrease tremors. Octanoic acid, also known as "caprylic acid," is a component in some foods, including coconut and its products (coconut milk and coconut oil), cow's milk (full-fat), peanut butter, and palm oil. No studies have yet been done looking at tremor levels in people who eat diets rich in these foods. However, mice that were first given harmaline (see above) to cause tremors had much less tremor after taking octanoic acid than mice that did not get octanoic acid.[7] Please see the Research chapter in <u>Section 4</u> to learn more about octanoic acid as a possible treatment for ET.

Diets rich in foods that contain octanoic acid (coconuts, milk, peanut butter, and palm oil) may reduce tremor.

One final note regarding diet: as mentioned in <u>Section 1</u>, low levels of vitamins such as B12 and D are associated with tremors due to ET and Parkinson's disease (PD). So be sure that you regularly eat a balanced diet, consider taking a vitamin supplement that provides the recommended daily amounts of these vitamins, and consider having your vitamin levels checked by your doctor.

There are a number of herbs and herbal medicine treatments (also known as "herbal supplements") that have been reported, anecdotally, to decrease tremors. Many of these herbs are known to reduce anxiety or help with sleep, and one of the benefits of reduced anxiety and better sleep can be a decrease in tremor. You can take most of these herbs in pill form, in a liquid that can be mixed in drinks, or in a tea that you drink before bedtime. Teas and liquid versions are widely regarded as better ways to get more of the herbal medicine into your body.

It is important to note that these herbal medicines have not been scientifically proven to reduce tremors and are not approved by the FDA for the treatment of tremor.

CAUTION: Some herbal medicines can be dangerous to take with other medicines your doctor gives you.[8] If you decide to try any of these, then please do so carefully and under the supervision of your doctor. You can check common ways herbs and medicines affect each other on the Natural Medicines Comprehensive Database website (http://naturaldatabase.thera-peuticresearch.com/home.aspx?Aspx-AutoDetectCookieSupport=1).Manyherbs can cause side effects. If you start to have side effects, it is best to stop taking the herbal medicine immediately and go see your doctor. Many of these herbs have also not been studied for use in pregnant women—so if you are pregnant, please talk to your doctor before taking any herbal medicine.

Valerian

Valerian is a flowering plant that is very fragrant and is one of the most widely used natural methods to improve sleep. In general, people who take valerian find that they have better quality sleep and can fall asleep faster.[9] Valerian is known to increase the amount of GABA, a chemical in the brain that is often low in people with ET. It is possible that this is how valerian helps to reduce tremors.

Skullcap

Skullcap is a flowering plant with blue and purple flowers that grows in the woods or wild meadows. It has been shown to help with anxiety and may even help to prevent neurological conditions like PD and Alzheimer's disease.[10]

Kava kava

Kava kava is a tall shrub that grows in the Pacific islands (such as Hawaii and Fiji). It is generally used as a sleep aid and muscle relaxant. Be careful when using this herb, as it often has a side effect similar to drinking alcohol. It also can cause liver damage, so you should not use kava kava if you have liver problems.[11]

Passionflower

Passionflower is a flowering vine with blue and bright pink flowers that grows in parts of America and in Europe.[12] It is used as a sleep aid and to treat anxiety. It is considered to be milder than valerian. A recent study[13] found that most people had lower anxiety levels after they took passionflower for four weeks.

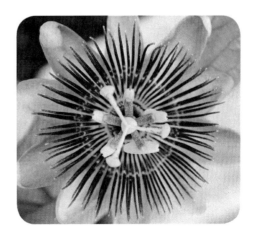

Corydalis

Corydalis is a plant with bright purple and blue flowers that grows in China. It is used to treat chronic pain.[14] Corydalis may work by increasing levels of dopamine, a chemical that is abnormally low in people with PD, in the brain. More research needs to be done to know if corydalis helps tremors due to ET as well as PD.[15]

Lavender

Lavender is a shrub from the Mediterranean that produces fragrant blue-violet flowers. It has a wide variety of uses, including as a sleep aid and as a treatment for anxiety, depression, headaches, and fatigue. In addition to its use in teas and supplements, lavender is one of the more common essential oils.[16]

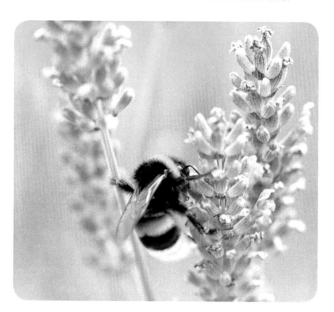

Chamomile

Chamomile is a tiny, daisy-like flower that grows in Europe, North Africa, and parts of Asia. It is most well known as a calming tea.[17] It is used for many purposes, including as a sleep aid, to treat anxiety and muscle spasms, to clear up skin rashes, and to help with digestion. It even may help treat certain infections. Studies suggest that chamomile may work by changing the way GABA (a chemical low in people with ET) works in the brain.[18,19] This may explain chamomile's helpful effect on tremors.

Combined supplements

Sometimes I am asked about herbal supplements that combine several of the above herbs. One of the more popular of these is Tremanol, which contains B vitamins, skullcap, passionflower, and valerian. Such combined supplements may help some people. In general, it is often more effective to take each herb separately in its pure form. This is because certain herbs need to be prepared in special ways that may not be possible in the combined supplement. You can still take more than one herb at the same time, as long as you do not have any medical conditions that would make it unsafe to do so. Always talk to your doctor before taking combined supplements or many separate herbs together.

BRANDS OF HERBAL SUPPLEMENTS

Patients often ask me what brand of herbal supplements is best. There are many choices. Generally, the purer the supplement, with fewer additives (extra ingredients), the better it should work.

The United States Pharmacopeial Convention keeps a list of vitamin and herbal supplement companies that volunteer to have their products tested for purity. You can find a current list of brands that submit to such testing on their website (www.usp.org/verification-services/program-participants).

Nature's Bounty is one such brand and offers valerian[20] supplements and chamomile and lavender essential oils.[21] Natural Factors has a kava kava supplement,[22] and Nature's Way offers non-GMO skullcap.[23] Herb Farm offers a non-GMO passionflower supplement.[24] You may want to go to a Chinese herbal store to purchase corydalis.

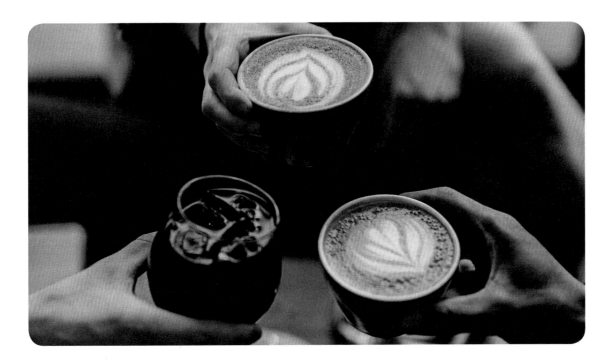

As described in Section 1, caffeine and alcohol can have mixed effects on tremor. Their effects depend on how much you drink and over what period of time. Not everyone is affected in the same way by these substances. Below are general ways in which caffeine and alcohol may affect ET.

Day to day

Caffeine in large doses (amounts) may make tremors worse

Alcohol in small doses may improve tremors

Over several years

Caffeine in low doses taken regularly may protect your brain and improve ET and PD tremor

Alcohol in high doses over time may damage your brain and make tremors worse

NOTE: If you do not currently drink alcohol, it is not recommended that you start drinking as a way to control your tremor.

Keep in mind that some people do not notice any difference in their tremors on a day-to-day basis after having caffeine or alcohol. Also, remember that caffeine is in foods such as chocolate as well as in drinks such as coffee, tea, soda, and energy drinks.

Dietary changes that may reduce your tremor include the following:

Have MORE	Have LESS
Baked or raw foods	Fried foods
Vegetables	Processed sugar
Olive and palm oils	Red meat
Coconuts	Caffeine
Nuts, nut butters	Large amounts of alcohol
Fish and cured meats	
Vitamin and herbal supplements (optional)	

REFERENCES

1. Scarmeasa N, Louis ED. Mediterranean diet and essential tremor. a case-control study. *Neuroepidemiology*. 2007;29(3-4):170-177.

2. Aharon-Peretz J, Badarny S, Ibrahim R, Gershoni-Baruch R, Hassoun G. Essential tremor prevalence is low in the Druze population in northern Israel. *Tremor Other Hyperkinet Mov (N Y)*. 2012;2:tre-02-81-390-1.

3. Berlin I, Grimaldi A, Landault C, Cesselin F, Puech AJ. Suspected postprandial hypoglycemia is associated with beta-adrenergic hypersensitivity and emotional distress. *J Clin Endocrinol Metab*. 1994;79(5):1428-33.

4. Louis ED, Zheng W, Mao X, Shungu DC. Blood harmane is correlated with cerebellar metabolism in essential tremor: a pilot study. *Neurology*. 2007;69(6):515-20.

5. Louis ED, Keating GA, Bogen KT, et al. Dietary epidemiology of essential tremor: meat consumption and meat cooking practices. *Neuroepidemiology*. 2008;30:161-166.

6. Louis ED, Factor-Litvak, Gerbin M, et al. Blood harmane, blood lead, and severity of hand tremor: evidence of additive effect. *Neurotoxicology*. 2011;32(2):227-32.

7. Nahab FB, Handforth A, Brown T, et al. Octanoic acid suppresses harmaline-induced tremor in mouse model of essential tremor. *Neurotherapeutics*. 2012;9(3):635-638.

8. Carrasco MC, Vallejo JR, Pardo-de-Santayana M, Peral D, Martín MA, Altimiras J. Interactions of Valeriana officinalis L. and Passiflora incarnata L. in a patient treated with lorazepam. *Phytother Res.* 2009;23(12):1795-6.

9. Bent S, Padula A, Moore D, et al. Valerian for sleep: a systematic review and meta-analysis. *Am J Med.* 2006;119(12):1005-1012.

10. University of Maryland Medical Center. Skullcap. Complementary and Alternative Medicine Guide. https://www.umm.edu/health/medical/altmed/herb/skullcap. Reviewed January 1, 2017.

11. University of Maryland Medical Center. Kava kava. Complementary and Alternative Medicine Guide. https://www.umm.edu/health/medical/altmed/herb/kava-kava. Reviewed January 1, 2017.

12. University of Maryland Medical Center. Passionflower. Complementary and Alternative Medicine Guide. https://www.umm.edu/health/medical/altmed/herb/passionflower. Reviewed January 1, 2017.

13. Villet S, Vacher V, Colas A, et al. Open-label observational study of the homeopathic medicine Passiflora Compose for anxiety and sleep disorders. *Homeopathy.* 2016;105(1):84-91.

14. Zhang Y, Wang C, Wang L, et al. A novel analgesic isolated from a traditional Chinese medicine. *Curr Biol.* 2014;24:117-23.

15. GaBi. 10 Natural Remedies for Essential Tremor. Health & Love Page website. https://healthandlovepage.com/10-natural-remedies-for-essential-tremor-in-hands. Published October 22, 2015.

16. University of Maryland Medical Center. Lavender. Complementary and Alternative Medicine Guide. https://www.umm.edu/health/medical/altmed/herb/lavender. Reviewed January 2, 2015.

17. University of Maryland Medical Center. German chamomile. Complementary and Alternative Medicine Guide. https://www.umm.edu/health/medical/altmed/herb/german-chamomile. Reviewed March 25, 2015.

18. Rodriguez-Fragoso L, Reyes-Esparza J, Burchiel S, Herrera-Ruiz D, Torre E. Risks and benefits of commonly used herbal medicines in México. *Toxicol Appl Pharmacol.* 2008;227(1):125-35.

19. Avallone R, Zanoli P, Puia G, Kleinschnitz M, Schreier P, Baraldi M. Pharmacological profile of apigenin, a flavonoid isolated from Matricaria chamomilla. *Biochem Pharmacol.* 2000;59:1387-1394.

20. Nature's Bounty. Nature's Bounty Valerian Root. https://www.naturesbounty.com/our-products/specialty/diet-supplements/valerian-root-plus-calming-blend-450-mg-100-capsules.

21. Nature's Bounty Earthly Elements. Our Products. http://www.earthlyelements.com.

22. Natural Factors. Stress-Relax Kava Kava. https://naturalfactors.com/product/kava-kava.

23. Nature's Way. Scullcap Herb. http://www.naturesway.com/Product-Catalog/Scullcap-Herb-100-Caps.

24. Herb Pharm. Passionflower. https://www.herb-pharm.com/products/product-detail/passionflower.

Did you know that there are many tools that can make daily life easier for people with tremors? These tools are often called "adaptive," because they are everyday products that are modified for people with tremor or other movement issues. Below I describe different items that can help you with activities like eating and drinking, writing, using your computer, getting dressed, getting in the door faster, and even making your hobbies easier! For each activity, I also describe small changes you can make that will help lessen your tremor and let you do more of the things you want to do.

My descriptions of specific tools below are based on my patients' experiences with these or similar products. The table at the end of this chapter lists these tools and the websites on which you can find them. Many of these products are also available through Amazon and other sellers, but I have tried to list the sellers with the lowest prices at the time of this publication. You may find these products at a lower price on other websites or in medical supply stores, so be sure to search around.

This is not a complete list of all the products available from all companies, and products that work for some people may not work for others. My blog on www.helpfortremors.com features up-to-date products and services as they come out. If you have tried something and found it to be particularly helpful, please leave a comment on the website to let me know about it!

NOTE: If you see an occupational therapist (OT) (see Section 3), he or she often has, or can get, many of these products for you to test out when you go in for an appointment. Your OT can also make recommendations for products that would be the most helpful to you.

EAT AND DRINK WITH FEWER SPILLS

There are a number of kitchen items that can make it easier for you to eat foods like soup and peas and to drink with fewer spills.

Weighted utensils and easy grip utensils

Weighted utensils include spoons, forks, and knives with special weights inside their handles. Certain knives, known as "rocker knives," can make it easier to cut most foods.

Weighted silverware may help you spill your food less by making you shake less.[1] Researchers do not completely understand how this works. Some believe the extra weight "distracts" your muscles by making them focus more on holding the extra weight than on picking up food. Being distracted can make you feel less stressed, which in turn can make your tremor better (see Section 1). Other researchers think the extra weight may put pressure on your muscles and nerves, which changes the signals they send to and get from your brain. The changed signals could then make your tremors decrease.[1]

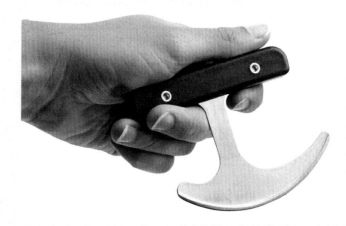

Photo credit: The Wright Stuff, Inc. www.wrightstuff.biz

Keep in mind that weighted utensils do not work for everybody. In some cases, especially if you have very weak arm or hand muscles, the extra weight may make it harder for you to hold a spoon or fork and could make your tremors worse. Some companies will allow you to return these items if you try them and they do not work for you.

Easy-grip utensils are another choice to help you eat more easily. They have either a larger handle or material on the handle that makes it less likely to slip out of your hand. One example is a soup bowl with a handle and a non-skid base.

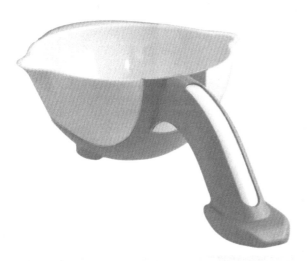

Photo credit: The Wright Stuff, Inc. www.wrightstuff.biz

LiftwareSteady™

If you have hand tremor that is caused by ET or Parkinson's disease, Liftware Steady can help you keep more food on your spoon or fork. Studies have shown that this device can help reduce shaking while eating by about 70 percent.[2] Liftware Steady has an electronic handle that senses your hand tremor and then moves in the opposite direction of your tremor. As a result, your utensil shakes less! It works with special utensil attachments, the most common of which is a regular spoon. There are also attachments for a soup spoon, fork, and spork. It uses a rechargeable battery and will last for an hour on a single charge.

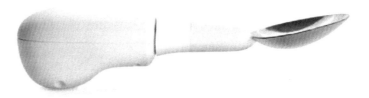

Verily Life Sciences https://liftware.com

SUGGESTIONS

Below are a few suggestions to make eating and drinking easier.[3,4] If you are eating at a restaurant, you can usually ask your server to make some of these changes for you.

- Eat soup from a mug rather than a bowl
- Eat with a spoon rather than a fork
- Keep your elbows close to your body or rest your arm on the edge of the table
- Fill drink cups halfway
- Use a straw to drink and a cup with a lid
- Carry a glass by holding it near the top instead of the bottom

Special pens, wrist weights or weighted gloves, and computer software can make it easier to write clearly and use your computer without double- or triple-tapping keys. Some of the software will work on a tablet or cell phone in addition to a computer.

Weighted pens

In the same way that weighted silverware can help your tremor, pens with weights on them can decrease your tremor so that it is easier to write more clearly. There are a variety of these pens on the market. You may need someone to put on the weights for you, as they are attached with screws. Some pens have wider bases that make it easier to write, as well, such as Steady Write pens. These are most helpful when writing on a smooth surface, like a desk, rather than on a notepad.

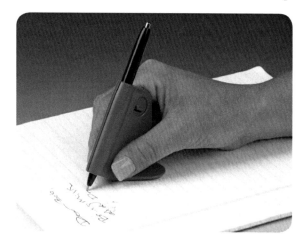

Photo credit: The Wright Stuff, Inc. www.wrightstuff.biz

Weighted gloves or wrist cuffs

If you have more severe tremors, weighted gloves or wrist cuffs may give you a little more support. These are meant to be worn while you are writing or typing. Some people find these help them eat more easily as well.[5]

The GyroGlove™ is a product in development that uses technology from satellites and rockets to counterbalance your tremor. It is a small device that attaches to a lightweight glove on your hand with a harness. This product is expected to be available by the end of 2018/early 2019.[6]

Computer software and accessories

Several companies have developed computer software and hardware that helps you avoid hitting extra keys on your keyboard or making extra clicks when using your computer mouse.

SteadyMouse is a Windows-based software platform that "detect[s] and remove[s] shaking motion before it reaches your cursor, and block[s] accidental clicks."[7] The company offers lower prices on a case-by-case basis if you cannot afford the full price.

SuperKeys is an affordable product from the UK that creates a special virtual keyboard on your Apple tablet or cell phone. The keyboard groups keys into seven sections and has intelligent word prediction and customizable keyboard shortcuts that help you get your point across with less frustration.[8]

The BigKeys LX Keyboard and keyguards provide larger keys and a keyboard cover to decrease extra keystrokes. They work with both Macintosh and Windows computers.[9]

Dictaphone software such as Dragon[10] allows you to speak words into your computer that the software will transcribe or "write out" into Microsoft Word, Google Docs, and even your email. Some Dragon products will also work with your mobile devices.

SUGGESTIONS

Here are a few suggestions to help make writing and using your computer easier:[3,4]

- Keep your elbows close to your body while writing or typing on a computer
- Rest your arm or wrist on a table while writing or typing
- Consider using a signature stamp
- Use voice commands on your phone or computer to text or email
- Set up your bills for automatic online payment so you do not have to write as many checks

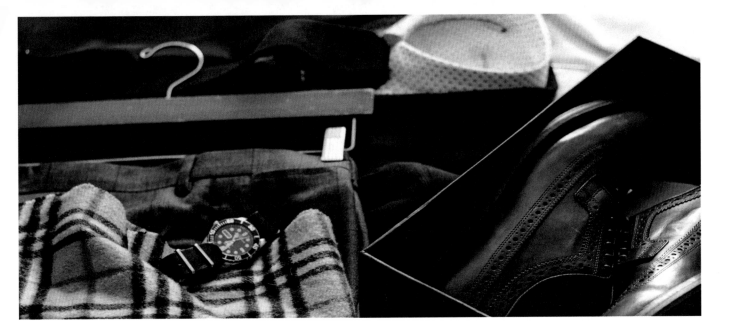

GET DRESSED AND GET IN THE DOOR FASTER

There are a few tools available to help you button your buttons, zip your zippers, and tie your shoes more easily. Several companies carry these "adaptive dressing aids."

A button hook is a wire loop you place over a button to help pull it through a buttonhole. A zipper pull is a small hook that attaches to the opening in your zipper tab. This gives you more to hold on to when you are zipping a zipper.

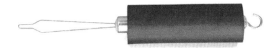

The Wright Stuff, Inc. www.wrightstuff.biz

Elastic shoe laces, which stay tied and simply stretch when you put on your shoes, magnetic belts, and jewelry clasps are other tools that may also help you get dressed more easily.

Getting a key in a lock or even turning some door knobs can be challenging with tremor. There are a few products that make this easier, as well.

A key turner fits around the base of your house key and gives you a longer and wider surface to grip, making it easier to get your key into the lock.

Door knob extenders and door knob grippers can also help by providing longer or "stickier" door handles that you can grab to open your doors.

SUGGESTIONS

The following suggestions, in combination with the tools described above, should help you get dressed and get in the door more easily.[3,4]

- Tighten your belly muscles when you are trying to get dressed and open doors
- Consider pants with elastic waists, pullover blouses, and slip-on shoes
- For shaving, use an electric razor
- Use a long-handled hairbrush or comb
- Keep your elbows close to your body when using a key or turning a door knob

So many patients have told me over the years that one of the things that bothers them most about having tremor is being unable to do the hobbies they love. This is hard for anyone with tremor. It is particularly hard for people who are retired and have a lot of free time to enjoy their hobbies. Further, one of the reasons people have hobbies is to help them relax. As I have described many times in this book, relaxing and lowering your stress levels will help you reduce your tremors. So, below are several adaptive tools and tips that may help you enjoy your hobbies again. Not all of these were created for people with tremor, but you may still find them useful.

Painting and drawing

I have always found it interesting that so many people with tremor are also artists. Drawing, painting, and other forms of visual art take a great deal of skill to develop. These hobbies also give the people who do them a great sense of accomplishment. I am blessed to have several pieces of art in my home and office drawn or painted by patients I have treated with deep brain stimulation (DBS) surgery. I hope that those of you who are artists are able to use these tools so you can continue to create your works of art.

A leaning bridge is an acrylic shelf that allows you to rest your hands and wrists so you can draw straighter lines and avoid smearing and smudging your work.

A mahl stick attaches to an easel and allows you to rest your hand so it is steady while you draw or paint.

Another option is to use a magnetic easel in combination with a lightly magnetized wrist or arm "glove." This idea was developed by researchers at Duke University specifically to help artists with tremors.[11]

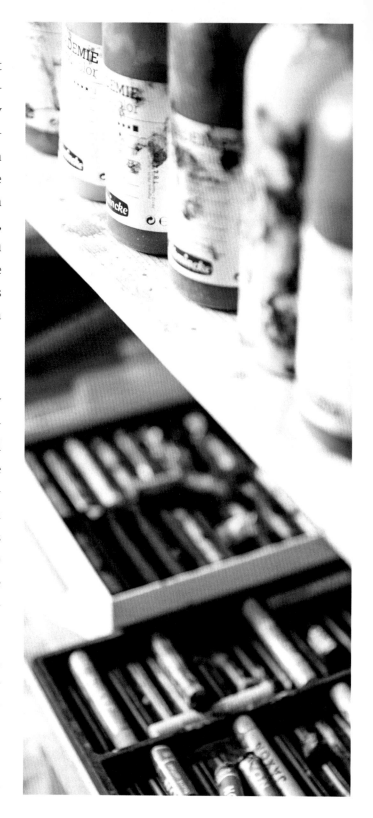

This post on the National Tremor Foundation website is written by an artist and offers helpful suggestions to other artists with tremor: www.tremor.org.uk/having-et-doesnt-stop-you-being-and-artist.html.

Golfing

Many of my patients with tremor often ask me if they will be "good golfers" after DBS surgery. To answer that question, I usually ask them if they were good golfers before they developed tremor! In all seriousness, tremor can significantly impact your ability to play golf, especially your putting ability. Some resources that are designed to improve putting skills in all golfers may also help golfers with tremor.

Mallet-style putters or putters with high MOIs ("moments of inertia") can help people with inconsistent putting as well as people with tremor. A counterbalanced putter (with added weight) may help reduce your tremor during putting, in the same way that weighted utensils and writing instruments can reduce tremor.

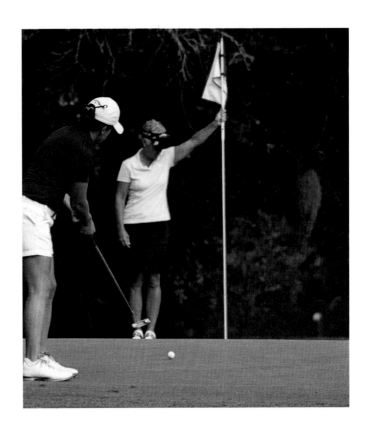

Many sports psychologists recommend you create a "pre-shot routine" that includes breathing and specific physical exercises you do before making a putt. One such professional has successfully helped a patient with ET (who does not take any medications to control his tremor) significantly improve his putting. Read his story here: www.womensgolf.com/stop-your-hands-shaking.

KNITTING AND CROCHETING

Knitting and crocheting can be a nightmare—and dangerous!—if you have tremors.

The Knitting Aid and the Knitting Aid Lite are devices that hold your knitting needles in place while you knit, making it easier to knit with tremors. The system works with a variety of different knitting needles.[12]

Kroh's Crochet Aid[13] may help make crocheting with tremors a little bit easier.

You can find many other assistive tools and tips for small changes to the way you do things on the International Essential Tremor Foundation website (**www.essentialtremor.org**).

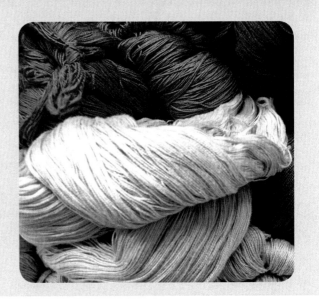

CHAPTER SUMMARY

Below is table of assistive tools, current costs, and websites on which you may purchase them. All products and pricing are based on what was available at the time of publication of this book in March 2018. As mentioned above, many of these products are available from multiple websites. I do not endorse any particular product, company, or website.

Product	Website	Cost
EATING AND DRINKING		
Weighted utensils	https://www.wrightstuff.biz/weutsetof4.html	$39.99/ set of 4
Rocker knife	https://www.wrightstuff.biz/rocking-t-knife.html	$18.95
Stay Bowl	https://www.maddak.com/stay-bowl-whitelight-gray-p-28256.html	$13.25
Scooper Plate	https://www.elderstore.com/scooper-plate-with-non-skid-base.aspx	$7.95
LiftwareSteady™	https://www.liftware.com/steady	$195.00 starter kit
WRITING		
Weighted pens	https://www.elderstore.com/weighted-universal-holder-for-pens-and-pencils.aspx	$20.95- $22.95
Steady Write Pen	https://www.wrightstuff.biz/steadywritepen.html	$9.95
Weighted glove	https://www.caregiverproducts.com/weighted-hand-writing-glove.html	$19.95
GyroGlove™	https://gyrogear.co (available end 2018/2019)	TBD
COMPUTER/PHONE USE		
SteadyMouse (Windows computer)	https://www.steadymouse.com	$43-$127
SuperKeys (Apple mobile)	https://www.cricksoft.com/us/superkeys	$12.99
BigKeys LX Keyboard (Mac/Windows)	https://www.ablenetinc.com/technology/computer-tablet-access/bigkeys-lx-keyboard	$149.00
BigKey LX keyguard	https://www.ablenetinc.com/bigkeys-lx-rigid-keyguard	$89.00
Dragon software	https://www.amazon.com/Dragon-NaturallySpeaking-Home-13-0-English/dp/B00LX4BZAQ	$41.84

Product	Website	Cost
GETTING DRESSED		
Button hook/ zipper pull	https://www.wrightstuff.biz/texture-grip-button-zipper-aid.html	$7.95- $14.95
Elastic shoelaces	https://www.wrightstuff.biz/black-elastic-shoelaces.html	$7.95
GETTING IN THE DOOR		
Key turners	https://www.wrightstuff.biz/keyturners.html	$3.95-$9.95
Doorknob grips	https://www.wrightstuff.biz/knob-switch-turners.html	$5.95 - $9.95
Doorknob extenders	https://www.healthykin.com//p-1356-lever-door-knob-extender.aspx	$14.95
HOBBIES		
Painting		
Acrylic shelf/ leaning bridge	https://www.amazon.com/Creative-Mark-Artists-Leaning-Bridge/dp/B004XMDFK8	$39.99
Mahl stick	http://www.jerrysartarama.com/art-paints/painting-supplies/mahl-sticks	$13.59-$31.99
Golf		
Putter counterweights	https://www.dickssportinggoods.com/p/superstroke-counter-core-weight-and-wrench-kit-15sutu50grmwghtnscmp	$9.99
Knitting		
Knitting Aid	https://www.knittingaid.com	$99.99
Crocheting		
Kroh's Crochet Aid	https://www.accesstr.com/Kroh-s-Crochet-Aid-p/kc01.htm	$15.95

REFERENCES

1. Lakie M, Walsh EG, Wright GW. Passive mechanical properties of the wrist and physiological tremor. *J Neurol Neurosurg Psychiatry*. 1986;49:669–676.

2. Pathak A, Redmond JA, Allen M, Chou KL. A noninvasive handheld assistive device to accommodate essential tremor: a pilot study. *Mov Disord*. 2014;29(6):838-42.

3. International Essential Tremor Foundation. Coping Tips for Everyday Living. IETF website. https://www.essentialtremor.org/coping/coping-tips-for-everyday-living.

4. Floyd J. An Occupational Therapy Perspective. IETF website. http://www.essentialtremor.org/coping/coping-with-et-articles/an-occupational-therapy-perspective.

5. McGruder J, Cors D, Tiernan AM, Tomlin G. Weighted wrist cuffs for tremor reduction during eating in adults with static brain lesions. *Am J Occup Ther*. 2003;57:507-516.

6. GyroGear. Frequently Asked Questions. http://gyrogear.co.

7. SteadyMouse. The SteadyMouse Project. https://www.steadymouse.com.

8. Crick Software. SuperKeys: The Assistive Keyboard for iPad and iPhone. http://www.cricksoft.com/us/superkeys.

9. AbleNet. BigKeys LX Keyboard. https://www.ablenetinc.com/technology/computer-tablet-access/bigkeys-lx-keyboard.

10. Nuance Communications. Dragon Speech Recognition Software. https://www.nuance.com/dragon.html.

11. Duke University. Artist's Easel with Arm Stabilizing Devices. Assistive Technology Design Projects website. https://sites.duke.edu/atdesign/2012/10/10/artists-easel-with-arm-stabilizing-devices. Published October 10, 2012.

12. Knitting Aid. https://www.knittingaid.com.

FINDING SUPPORT FROM OTHERS WHO SHAKE

You may not realize that there is support out there for people with tremors. You are not alone. There are a number of ways you can connect with other people who have tremors. Below I describe many ways that you can get support from others and places you can go to get reliable information about tremors and treatments.

SUPPORT GROUPS

Local support groups

Local support groups are meetings led by a person who has tremors, a physician, or a combination of both. The meetings may be sponsored by an organization, like the International Essential Tremor Foundation (IETF), or by a hospital system. These wonderful meetings serve two purposes. First, they connect you with other people who have tremors. Second, they provide you with information about tremors and ways to help stop or reduce them.

I co-led a support group for years, and I found that one of its greatest benefits was that people with tremors could connect with others just like them. At meetings, you can talk to other people about your experiences and learn from them about theirs. You can share struggles you are having, and as you do, you will realize that other people are struggling with the same things. You can share ideas that have helped you with your tremors, and learn new ideas from others.

Often, support groups will bring in experts to talk about different areas. In the essential tremor (ET) support group that I co-led, we brought in movement disorder neurologists to talk about the causes of tremors, different ways tremors affect people's lives, and medicines that are used to treat tremors. Sometimes I would speak, as a neurosurgeon, about surgical treatments for tremors and about the latest research. These support groups are great resources. The information is the most up to date, and the format lets you ask an expert direct questions. We even had support group members who would showcase their talents by singing, playing a musical instrument, or reading poetry. The talent in the group I led was amazing!

I co-led this group with a man named Eric who has ET. This team, of a person with ET and a doctor who treats ET, was very helpful for the group. Eric did a wonderful job helping plan meetings, making sure we focused on topics important to people with ET, and sharing feedback from the group about issues people were not comfortable telling a doctor. For example, a couple of people from our support group also went to one of our "patient events" (see section below). They mentioned to Eric after the event that they were bothered by one of our neurologist's presentations, which showed videos of patients with ET. They said the videos were too long and made them uncomfortable to watch for more than a few seconds. This feedback was priceless, because we were able to change future videos. We as doctors learned that people with ET wanted us to focus more on outcomes after treatment and give people a vision of what could be rather than what is. Just as Eric brought a great deal to the group from a patient's point of view, as a doctor I was able to help arrange speakers and provide information.

To find out where there may be a support group in your area, visit the IETF or National Tremor Foundation (NTF) website. These sites list any support group that has been registered with their organizations and will often post meeting locations and dates. You can also ask your neurologist about support groups in the area.

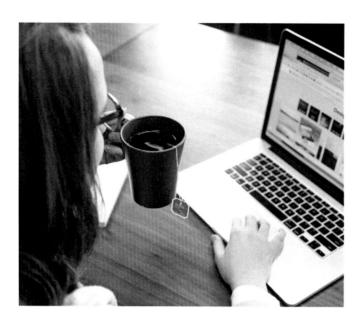

Social media pages and groups

These days, social media is a fantastic way to connect people with similar interests. As you search through social media sites such as Facebook, you will find numerous "pages" for people with tremors. Some of these are sponsored by organizations, such as the IETF or NTF, while others are managed by people like you who have tremors. These sites provide information including dates and times of support group meetings, tips for managing your tremors, the latest news about treatments, and insurance coverage issues for newer therapies. I created a Facebook page, "Help for Tremors" where I post updates on many of the topics in this book. It is also a place where people with tremors can post comments or questions to which I will respond. There are also many groups on social media, some public and some private, that serve as an online support groups in which you can share your stories, discuss concerns you have, or share tips that have helped you.

Starting a support group

While support groups have become more popular in recent years and many are available, there are some areas that do not yet offer support groups. So how can you start one? Well, the good news is, anyone can start a support group! If you contact the IETF or go to their website (www.essentialtremor.org), they

will train you to be a support group leader and give you information that you can pass out at meetings. They will also give you free advertising on their website for your meetings.

For meeting locations, you have several options. Your local chamber of commerce may have a listing of meeting spaces that can be reserved free of charge. Many apartment buildings or housing communities have a common room that can be reserved once each quarter for events. You can also talk to your neurologist about using meeting spaces connected to doctors' offices or hospitals. For our support group meetings, we used a conference room connected to one of our medical facilities after hours. Using this type of space has the added benefit of getting your neurologist interested in helping you run the group, provide content for the meetings, or both.

You likely will want to host your support group meetings on Tuesday or Wednesday evenings. Meetings work well between 6:30 and 8:30 pm. As the meetings are often during dinner hours, it is helpful to provide a light snack (such as sandwiches) and bottled drinks for your guests. Don't forget the straws! Depending on the size of your group, you may wish to have different members bring in food and drinks for different meetings. If you have a large group, you can ask your neurologist to see whether the office/hospital system will provide funding for snacks, or whether a medical company that makes products for tremor patients will sponsor your group.

The format of your meetings can vary from informal conversations to more formal presentations by doctors, occupational therapists, or researchers. Most support groups meet quarterly, but you can adjust the schedule based on the needs of your group. Keep track of contact information, such as email addresses, for those who attend your group, so you can send reminders about meetings. You also may want to start a social media page and group so your members can connect with one other between meetings.

Health chats

Some doctors' offices or hospitals will sponsor online "chats" with a neurologist or a neurosurgeon. The doctor will answer questions you submit to a website either in advance or live during a half-hour to one-hour broadcast. These chats may occur every year or sporadically, because doctors and hospitals often set them up to get more business. The information provided in these chats can be very helpful. The questions asked in advance are usually grouped by topic, and the doctor answers the most frequently asked questions first.

You will log on to a website during the chat and will be able to read people's questions and the doctor's answers. These chats are often in written format, only because video sometimes slows down internet speed; however, sometimes the chat may come with video so you can see the doctor respond live. As you think of new questions during the broadcast, you will be able to send them in. Usually any questions the doctor does not answer before time runs out will be answered afterward and posted in the written transcript of the chat, which usually will be available on the doctor's or hospital's website.

Patient events

A doctor, hospital, or company sponsors patient events in order to advertise or market to increase business. These are usually half-day or full-day events, hosted on a Saturday in a large hotel conference room or similar facility. Typically, the events include several speakers, such as a neurologist, neurosurgeon, occupational therapist, and psychologist, who will talk about causes of and treatments for tremors. Sometimes, patients with tremors will be asked to speak about their personal experiences with tremors and treatments they have had (such as

deep brain stimulation). There may be a roundtable discussion forum as well, in which the audience can ask the speakers questions.

At patient events I have organized, we put out assistive products, like weighted utensils, for people to try. We also set up stations during breaks for people to get "mini assessments" to see how much tremor may be affecting their lives. After the screening, physician assistants would recommend whether people should see a movement disorder neurologist for more help. Of course, you need a formal exam by a qualified doctor to figure out the cause of your tremors and give you the best treatment plan. However, getting an idea of how much your tremor affects your life can be helpful. Sometimes you may even be able to schedule an appointment with a doctor at these events and avoid a long waiting list for appointments. As a side note, because a hospital or company sponsors these events, they also will provide food throughout the day.

FOUNDATIONS AND ASSOCIATIONS

International Essential Tremor Foundation (IETF)

The IETF is a nonprofit organization based in the US that provides information and resources to people with ET. They also support medical research by giving grants to people studying the causes of and new treatments for ET. Their website (www.essentialtremor.org) provides lots of information, including facts about ET, a brochure to help you tell the difference between tremors from ET and Parkinson's disease, information on how to cope with ET, various treatments for ET, and many other resources. There are links to assistive tools, such as zipper assists and weighted utensils, as well as links to books written about ET from a patient's point of view. You can also search for a movement disorder neurologist on their website, as well as learn about the latest research being done. As mentioned above, if you are looking for a support group meeting to attend, or are looking to start a support group, the IETF website has a lot of information on this, too.

National Tremor Foundation (NTF)

The NTF is an organization based in the United Kingdom that provides much of the same information and resources as the IETF. The NTF website (www.tremor.org.uk) also has a section in which people with ET tell their stories and discuss how ET has impacted their lives. This section is inspirational, as many of the stories are written by professionals who have kept going with their work in spite of their tremors. The stories also include some helpful "how-tos." For example, one story written by an artist describes workarounds he uses to keep his tremors from limiting his painting.

American Parkinson's Disease Association (APDA)

The APDA is an organization based in the US that provides information and resources for people with Parkinson's disease (PD). Their website (www.apdaparkinson.org) gives information about tremors and other symptoms specific to PD. They offer a webinar education series that focuses on different topics related to PD, and there is also a special section with resources for veterans with PD.

Michael J. Fox Foundation

The Michael J. Fox Foundation is an organization that supports research to find a cure for PD. The website (www.michaeljfox.org) provides information about tremors and other symptoms of PD and gives a long list of current research studies. There is also a large section with links to resources to learn more about PD and its treatment.

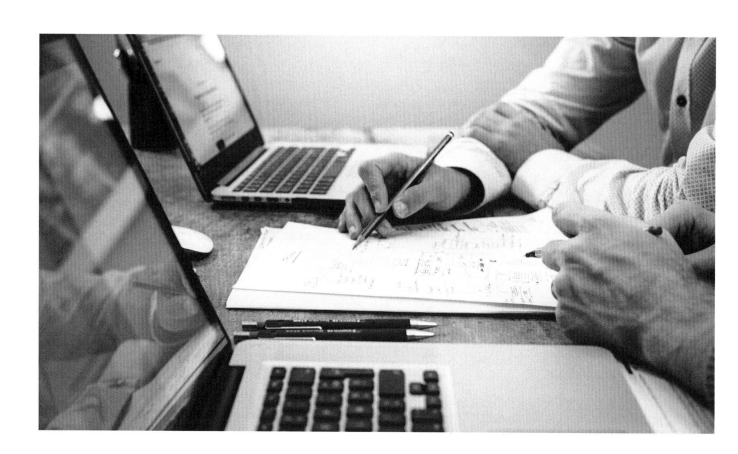

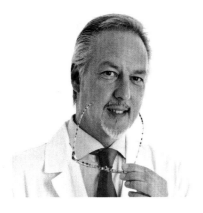
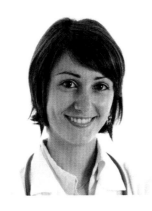
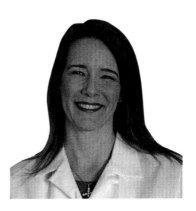
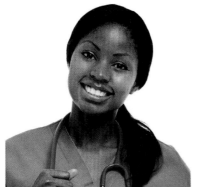
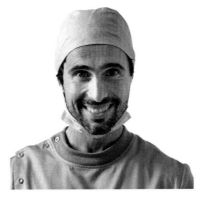
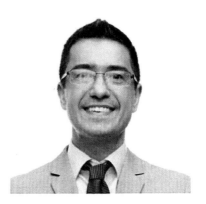
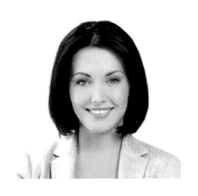
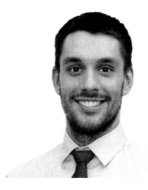
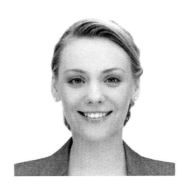

SECTION

3

MEDICAL AND SURGICAL OPTIONS

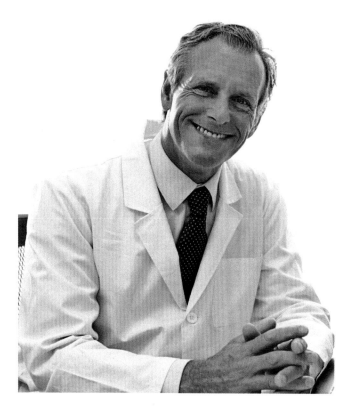

AT THE DOCTOR

Going to the doctor can be scary! I have noticed over my years of practicing neurosurgery that many patients have had the "shakes" for several years before ever coming to see a doctor. When I would ask why they waited so long, responses would vary from, "Well, I thought maybe it would just go away," to "I didn't realize how much it was affecting my life," to "I was afraid that a doctor would tell me something was wrong with me." I think fear has a lot to do with all of these answers. We have so many ideas running through our heads about what may be wrong with us. We search WebMD or Google and find all kinds of horrible diseases and illnesses that match our symptoms. The last thing we want is to have someone tell us that one of those horrible diseases is what is actually causing our problems.

Did you know doctors do this too? We actually are some of the worst offenders, because we have spent years learning about all the rare diseases that affect 0.0001% of the population. So when something goes "wrong" with us, we automatically think the cause will be the most horrible disease we can imagine, even though we are more likely to win a Powerball jackpot than to have that disease. We all avoid the doctor—but when we do, our fears often get worse. We may try to ignore them, and we may be successful for a while. But here's the thing: your subconscious keeps worrying even if you consciously choose to ignore something. So that fear will come out in other ways, and usually at really inconvenient times. (That is the topic of another book entirely!)

The best way to get over your fears is to get information. Information often makes fear powerless, so it is important to get the "right," good quality information. You can best get this directly from a medical professional. As I am neurosurgeon who has treated patients with tremors for over 10 years, this book is a good place to start. However, even this book is not a substitute for a visit to your doctor for an evaluation. Every situation and every person is different. Most of you will be able to use many of the techniques described in the first

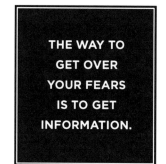

THE WAY TO GET OVER YOUR FEARS IS TO GET INFORMATION.

part of this book and significantly control your tremors. However, I still recommend you see a doctor about your tremors, because your doctor can give you information that is specific to you and your situation.

Many of you reading this book may find your shaking is due to essential tremor. Wouldn't it be great to hear that in person from a doctor? Think about the stress that would take off of you! You would know for certain that you are not dying of some horrible disease and that you have a benign (not life-threatening) condition with good treatment options available. That certainly would make me feel better. For those of you who have other conditions causing your tremors, getting information from your doctor is just that—information. As a patient, you always have the right to decide which treatments to have or refuse. I will tell you this many times in this section of the book: having information about the cause of your tremors can only help you. Once you have that information, you can learn about your options for treatment. And then you have the power to decide. When you take control, you take the power away from your fear.

To get you started with good quality information, this section will describe what to expect during your visits to the doctor, from your first visit onward. Knowing what to expect will help take away that fear of the unknown.

At the doctor's office, several things usually happen. You fill out paperwork, your doctor or an assistant asks you questions, and your doctor examines you. Then your doctor talks to you about what is causing your symptoms and makes recommendations about what you should do next. These recommendations may include having your blood drawn, having certain types of x-rays, or seeing another doctor or medical provider who can help you. I will explain what to expect during each of these parts of your visit with your doctor.

What to expect during your first doctor's visit:

- *Telling your doctor about yourself*
- *A medical exam by your doctor*
- *A discussion about what may be causing your problem*
- *Recommendations for next steps*
  - *Drawing your blood*
  - *Taking x-rays*
  - *Sending you to another doctor or medical professional*

"MEDICAL HISTORY," OR TELLING YOUR DOCTOR ABOUT YOURSELF

Giving a medical history simply means telling your doctor background information about yourself and your medical problems. This usually happens in two different ways. First, you likely will be asked to fill out a lot of paperwork. Then when you see your doctor, he or she will go over this information with you. Your doctor may ask you the same questions that you already answered in your paperwork. This may seem redundant to you, and in an ideal world this would not happen. However, depending on how the office staff handles paperwork, your doctor may not have seen the papers you filled out before your visit. Sometimes another staff member is using those papers to enter your information into a computer while you are seeing the doctor, so that the office has a permanent record of your information.

There are many background questions that you will be asked at the doctor. Below I break these down into different categories and include an explanation of why doctors ask you this information. This is a pretty long list! Keep in mind that sometimes you can fill out paperwork before your visit—either you receive it in the mail, or you fill it out on a computer. In the office, paperwork may take up to 30 minutes to fill out, so leave yourself time before your appointment if you did not fill out the paperwork in advance. When you review your information in person with the doctor, it can take anywhere from 10 to 30 minutes, depending on the number of problems you have or had in the past.

PERSONAL OR "DEMOGRAPHIC" INFORMATION

You will be asked your gender, age, and race. Some medical conditions occur more often in women than in men, as we see in essential tremor. Some conditions, such as Parkinson's disease, are more likely to occur at a certain age. And certain conditions, such as multiple sclerosis, are more common in people of a certain ethnicity.

WHY ARE YOU SEEING THE DOCTOR TODAY?

The first question you likely will be asked is, "Why are you seeing the doctor today?" This information becomes part of your "history of present illness," or "HPI," as you may hear or see on certain forms. When you see a doctor for your tremors, you will be asked all kinds of questions to help your doctor figure out what may be causing the tremors. Your doctor wants to hear from you at this point. He or she will see your tremor in person during your exam (described below). But your input on your experiences with the tremor is as important as what your doctor sees during the exam. It will help the doctor best "diagnose" you, or figure out what is causing your shaking.

Questions you will be asked:

- *What shakes? One arm, a hand, a finger? Both legs? Your head, voice, or whole body?*
- *Is your shaking barely noticeable or is it very obvious to anyone who is watching you?*
- *How old were you when you first noticed the shaking?*
- *When do you notice the shaking now? Do you notice it while eating or sitting still?*
- *How long does the shaking last when it happens?*
- *Does anything make the shaking better? Does anything make it worse?*
- *Do you notice anything else, like stiff arms or legs, or being off balance when you walk?*

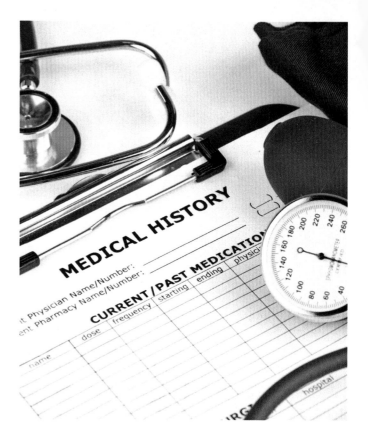

MEDICAL PROBLEMS

Your medical problems, or "past medical history," includes any health issue you have ever had, even if it is not a problem now. I often see patients leave this section blank or leave something out because nothing else is "bothering" them at the time of the visit or because the medical problem is under control with medicine. Leaving out information can make it harder for your doctor to figure out what is wrong with you and may lead to dangerous problems, particularly when ordering medicine for you or recommending certain treatments or surgeries.

So even if your blood pressure is "normal" now because you take medicine for it, it is important to mention to your doctor that you have had high blood pressure before. And if you have recovered completely from a previous stroke, be sure to mention that as well. Often on the paperwork you fill out there will be a list of different medical conditions you can check off. However, as mentioned above, your doctor may not have that list with him or her during your visit—so remember to mention your conditions again.

For a neurologist or neurosurgeon, it is most important to mention if you have or ever had:

- *A heart attack or problems with your heart not beating regularly or not pumping blood as it should*
- *Problems breathing, from asthma, COPD (chronic obstructive pulmonary disease), or other lung issues*
- *Easy bruising or a lot of bleeding after a cut or from a surgery*
- *Blood clots in your lungs, legs, or arms*
- *Problems with your brain, spinal cord, or nerves*
- *Any reason you have ever been in the hospital or emergency room*

SURGERIES

Your "past surgical history" includes any reason you have ever had surgery in the past. Have you had your gall bladder or appendix taken out? Have you had a heart bypass surgery or a stent put in? Have you ever had brain surgery? Did you ever have a knee or shoulder repaired, or a broken bone operated on? This information is important for a few reasons. First, in case you forget to mention medical problems you have had, your past surgeries may give your doctor an idea of your other problems. Second, during some surgeries you may have had metal pieces placed in your body. Your doctor needs to know about these, since some x-rays are not possible or safe to have if you have certain types of metal in your body.

MEDICINES

You will need to bring a list of your medicines to your doctor's appointment. This should include the name of the medicine, the "dose" (which is often listed in milligrams (mg)), and how often you take the medicine (once a day, every other day, etc.). You can also bring all of your pill bottles with you if you do not have a list. It generally is not a good idea to bring pills with you that are in pill boxes and not in their original bottles. It will be hard for your doctor to know what you are taking just by looking at the pill. It is a good idea to carry a list of your medicines and doses with you at all times and be sure your emergency contact has a copy of this list as well. In fact, if you do not have such a list, you should put down this book—make a list and put it in your wallet now.

Also make sure to write down anything you take on a regular basis, including non-prescription medicines, vitamins, and herbs. Some medicines or treatments your doctor prescribes may not be safe to take with other medicines and vitamins. It also is very important to mention any medicine you take that make your blood "thin," including Coumadin, Plavix, Eliquis, and others. Aspirin, Motrin or ibuprofen, and other over-the-counter pain medicines can make your blood thin as well. Mentioning these medicines is especially important if you are seeing a surgeon, even if it is just for a consultation.

Your medicine list should include:

- *Medicines any doctor has given you*
- *Over-the-counter medicines (Tylenol, Motrin, Aspirin, etc.)*
- *Vitamins*
- *Herbs*

> **IT IS A GOOD IDEA TO CARRY A LIST OF YOUR MEDICINES AND DOSES WITH YOU AT ALL TIMES AND BE SURE YOUR EMERGENCY CONTACT HAS A COPY OF THIS LIST AS WELL. YOU SHOULD PUT DOWN THIS BOOK NOW AND MAKE THIS LIST AND PUT IT IN YOUR WALLET IF YOU HAVEN'T DONE THAT BEFORE.**

Some people are "allergic" to certain medicines. This means that when they take a particular medicine, they have a bad "reaction" to it. In other words, something happens to a person that is not supposed to happen when taking that medicine. These reactions can range from feeling sick to your stomach or a headache, to rashes all over your body and difficulty breathing. There are certain allergic reactions that are more concerning to doctors than others.

Please tell your doctor if any of these things happen or have happened when taking a medicine:

- *Itching or a rash*
- *Hives or blisters on the skin*
- *Trouble breathing*
- *Swelling of your body or your tongue*
- *Throwing up and belly pain*

In this section of your medical history, it also is important to mention any reactions like this you have to foods, particularly shellfish. Some of the x-rays your doctor may want to order have to be done differently if you have a shellfish allergy. What you do not need to worry about mentioning here are environmental allergies, such as sniffling and coughing from dust, pollen, or animals.

Your doctor will want to know if you drink alcohol, smoke cigarettes, use marijuana, or take any drugs that have not been prescribed to you. Your doctor will ask how much you drink and how often, and how much you smoke and how long you have been smoking. If you have used drugs your doctor will ask what kind, how often, and when the last time was that you used them. It is very important to be truthful when answering these questions and to mention if you have done these things in the past, even if you do not do them now. Remember that your doctor is only trying to help you and to suggest treatments for you that will be safe. If you do not want to answer these questions on a form and would rather talk about them in person with the doctor, then write on the form: "Will discuss with doctor."

It is important to mention your alcohol use, because with certain conditions, your tremor could get better or worse with alcohol. As mentioned in the first section of this book, smoking can make your tremors worse. So your doctor may recommend ways to help you stop smoking. I discuss marijuana and its effect on tremor in the Research chapter of this book. If you use marijuana, your doctor will want to discuss this with you further. Some street drugs can cause problems if taken with certain medicines your doctor may want to give you.

FAMILY HISTORY

Some conditions that cause tremors run in families. Your doctor will ask you if anyone else in your family has tremors. It is most important to mention if anyone in your immediate family—including parents, grandparents, brothers and sisters, and children—has had tremors. If you also know what caused their tremors, then tell your doctor. If all you know is that your father had the "shakes," then that is okay, too. Your doctor will want to know how old any family members were when they first noticed their tremors. All of this information will help your doctor figure out what may be causing your tremors.

It is also important to mention any other major medical problems that people in your immediate family have had, including heart attacks (especially if they happened before age 40), strokes, breathing problems, and cancer.

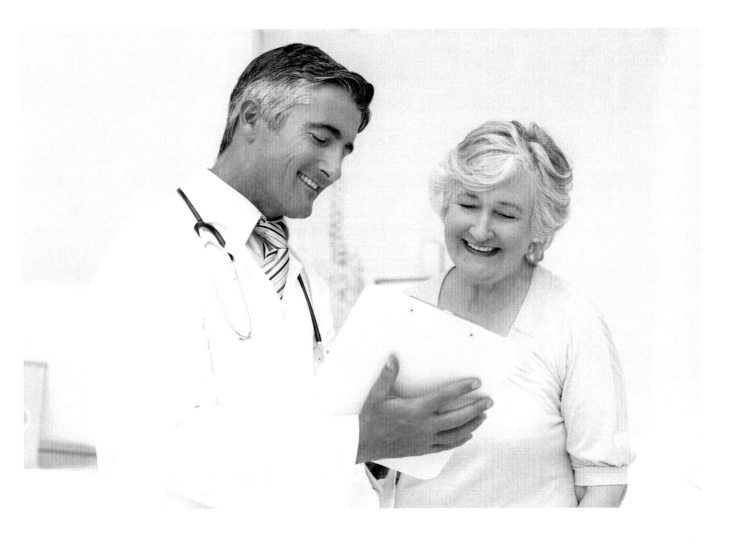

The last piece of medical history you will have to fill out during your doctor's visit will usually be a long list of questions about every organ system in your body. You will see questions about your brain, lungs, heart, kidneys, bowels, skin, etc. These questions serve two purposes. One is to make sure you have mentioned every medical problem you have, so that nothing is missed. The second is to find out if you currently have any other problems for which you may need to see a doctor.

When answer these screening questions, sometimes called a "review of systems," you should mention only those things that bother you all the time or have been bothering you recently. For example, if you have been coughing for two weeks, you would say "yes" to the question, "Have you been coughing?" However, if you had a cough six months ago due to a cold, you would answer "no" to that question.

Some screening items are especially important to mention during a visit with a neurologist or a neurosurgeon:

- *Fever or cough*
- *Chest pains*
- *Difficulty breathing*
- *Being off balance*
- *Seizures*
- *Bleeding problems*

If you are seeing a doctor for your tremors, you may be asked to fill out a form that asks you how much you feel your tremor affects your life. This form is often used as another screening tool to figure out whether you are likely to need some type of treatment for your tremor. Below I give an example of such a form and how it may be used. There are many different forms available, including an "official" and "validated" form from the International Essential Tremor Foundation (IETF).

Name: _____ DOB: ___/___/___ Date: ___/___/___

For each question below, please mark the box that best describes your current situation.

[N]   [S]   [A]

N: Never/No   S: Sometimes   A: All the time/Yes

HOW HAS YOUR TREMOR AFFECTED YOU PROFESSIONALLY?			
I have trouble doing my job.	N	S	A
I have changed jobs.	N	S	A
I retired early.	N	■	A
I can only work part time.	N	■	A
I am having financial trouble.	N	S	A
HOW HAS YOUR TREMOR AFFECTED YOUR LEISURE ACTIVITIES?			
I have lost interest in my hobbies.	N	■	A
I quit some of my hobbies.	N	■	A
I had to change or develop new hobbies.	N	■	A
I have trouble writing letters and completing forms.	N	S	A
HOW HAS YOUR TREMOR AFFECTED YOUR LIFESTYLE?			
I have trouble using a keyboard on a computer, or dialing a phone	N	S	A
I am unable to fix small things around the house (for example, change light bulbs, minor plumbing, fixing household appliances, fixing broken items).	N	S	A
* I have trouble with my personal hygiene (for example, brushing or flossing my teeth) and appearance (for example, buttoning, zipping, and tying shoes).	N	S	A
* I have trouble eating (for example, bringing food to mouth, spilling) and drinking liquids (for example, bringing to mouth, spilling, pouring).	N	S	A
HOW DOES YOUR TREMOR AFFECT YOU PERSONALLY?			
I am embarrassed by my tremor.	N	S	A
I am depressed.	N	S	A
I feel isolated or lonely.	N	S	A
I am nervous or anxious and I worry about the future.	N	S	A
I have difficulty concentrating.	N	S	A
* My tremor interferes with my relationships with my family, friends and/or coworkers.	N	S	A
* I use alcohol more frequently than I would like to.	N	S	A
Add the total points for each column			
Multiply each column's points by the appropriate number:	x0	x1	x2
Multiplied totals for each column			
Add the five multiplied columns totals together			

If the **total** number **exceeds 20**, or the patient answers **S, or A** to any 1 of the **starred questions**, please consider referral to a movement disorder neurologist

Now that you have answered all those questions—thank goodness!—your doctor will want to do a physical exam to see what your tremor looks like in person. You may or may not be asked to put on an "exam gown" for the physical exam. Most neurologists will ask you to do this for the first visit, because they want to be sure they are checking for ALL neurological problems, in addition to whatever may be causing your tremor. Also, sometimes the way the muscles in your arms or legs look can give your doctor a clue about what is causing your tremor. You can leave your undergarments on under the gown. In addition to the "general exam," neurologists will also do a neurological exam, which focuses mainly on your brain, spinal cord, and nerves. A neurosurgeon likely will not do a general exam unless he or she is planning to operate on you in the next few weeks.

The general exam includes listening to your heart and lungs with an instrument called a stethoscope. The doctor will place the stethoscope on your chest in a few different spots and ask you to breathe quietly. Then he or she will move the stethoscope around your chest and back and ask you to breathe deeply. Next, the doctor will have you lie down on the exam table and will push on your belly and may also listen to your belly with a stethoscope. These tests tell your doctor if you have any major medical problems for which you would need to see a different kind of doctor for treatment.

Next, I will describe the steps of the neurological exam in more detail and explain what your doctor is looking for.

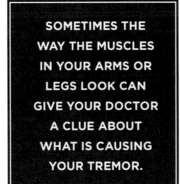

SOMETIMES THE WAY THE MUSCLES IN YOUR ARMS OR LEGS LOOK CAN GIVE YOUR DOCTOR A CLUE ABOUT WHAT IS CAUSING YOUR TREMOR.

A complete neurological exam usually takes between 10 and 20 minutes to complete. The exam does include questions—yes, more questions!—that will test your knowledge or ask you to remember certain things. But most of the exam will involve you moving your arms and legs in certain ways to test how strong you are and how easily you can feel a touch. Then you will be asked to do different tasks that may make your tremor more obvious.

Mental status

Neurological exams usually start with a test of your memory and thinking ability. This is called a "mental status exam." During this section, you will be asked to say things that you may consider silly, including your name, birthdate, your spouse's and children's names, and describing what you ate for breakfast or dinner. You will be asked to state the current date or season and your present location. You may be asked to name the President and Vice President of the United States, and you likely will be shown objects and asked to name them.

You will be asked to spell words forwards and backwards and to count down from 100 by threes or sevens. Your doctor may tell you three words, such as "dog, orange, 43," ask you to repeat them, and then ask you several minutes later if you can remember those words. Some of these questions can be difficult to answer, especially the math, spelling, and memory questions. Try not to get frustrated! The doctor asks these questions to help figure out what is causing your tremor, discover any other problems you may have, and figure out the best treatment for you. Many people with essential tremor (ET) and Parkinson's disease have some trouble with this part of the exam.

CRANIAL NERVES

"Cranial nerves" are nerves that come out of the base of your brain in the back of your head and control your ability to move your eyes, face, and head and to feel, taste, smell, see, hear, and a few other things. This is the part of the exam where your doctor will shine a light in your eyes, look in the back of your throat, and ask you to say, "Ahhhh." He or she will also ask you to look in different directions while keeping your head still, move your head in certain directions, and will test your hearing and ask if it feels normal when he or she touches your face. This is an important part of the exam to help your doctor figure out the cause of your tremors. Certain conditions that cause tremor also cause problems with the cranial nerves, but cranial nerves should work normally in people with ET.

Muscles

Your muscles work because your brain, spinal cord, and nerves tell them to work. Your brain has a thought that it wants to move your arm, for example, so it sends a message to your spinal cord, which sends a message to the nerves in your arm, which then tell your arm muscles to move. So testing the strength of your muscles can tell your doctor if there may be problems with your nerves, spinal cord, or brain. During this part of the exam, your doctor will ask you to use your arms to push against his or her arm or hand, and to use your arms to pull his or her arm or hand towards you. Your doctor will ask you to squeeze his or her hand tightly, and to spread your fingers out widely and hold them strongly. You will be asked to raise your knee up, kick backwards, and to push your feet down like you are pressing the gas pedal in a car and then point your toes back up to the ceiling. Having weaknesses in your muscles gives your doctor clues about the cause of your tremor. He or she will also test the stiffness or tightness of your muscles and will watch you walk down the hall or across the room. Stiffness or difficulty walking in combination with a tremor can be a sign that you have Parkinson's disease. Muscle strength and tone are usually normal in people with ET.

Sensation/Feeling

In addition to making your muscles move, your nerves also are the reason you can feel someone touching your hand, feel heat from a fire, or feel pain when you stub your toe. Your doctor will test your ability to feel different kinds of sensations, including gentle touch, a sharp pricking sensation (from the end of a broken cotton swab or tongue depressor), and vibration from a tuning fork, and your ability to know the positions of your fingers and toes with your eyes closed. Finally, your doctor will ask you to stand up and close your eyes. He or she will gently pull back your shoulders and see how well you can keep your balance. Don't worry—your doctor will not let you fall! As with the other parts of the neurological exam, results from the sensory exam give your doctor clues about your condition. Sensation is usually normal in patients with ET.

Reflexes

You know how your knee jumps when your doctor taps on it with the little hammer? That is called a reflex. Reflexes give doctors information about how your nerves are working. There are many reflexes other than the knee reflex all over the body, so expect your doctor to use the hammer to tap on the back of your ankle, the inside and outside of your elbow, your forearm, and sometimes even your jaw. (Usually the doctor puts a thumb on your jaw and taps that so it does not hurt as much!) Most people with ET have normal reflexes.

Darlene A Mayo MD FAANS   **STOP SPILLING YOUR SOUP!   The Complete Essential Tremor Solution**

Everything I've described to you above are the "standard" parts of the neurological exam. If you are seeing a doctor for tremors, then you will have some additional parts to your exam. These include placing your hands in your lap while the doctor looks for a tremor. If your hands shake when they are in your lap, this is called a "resting tremor." This is common in people with Parkinson's disease. You will also be asked to hold your hands out in front of you. If you shake with your arms extended, this is called "postural tremor." This is common in people with ET. You will be asked to do a variety of movements with your hands, which may include using your index (pointer) finger to touch your doctor's finger and then touch either your nose or your chin. (For people with more severe tremor, I have them touch their chins or their chests instead so they do not risk poking themselves in the eye.) You will be asked to do this a few times in a row.

You also may be asked to pour water from one cup to another over a sink, or to bring an empty cup up to and away from your mouth, as if you were drinking. If you shake during these tasks, it is called "intention tremor," which is the most common type of tremor you see in ET. This is what makes it hard to eat, drink, get a key in a door, write, and type on a keyboard. Lastly, you likely will be asked to try to draw a spiral on a paper without lifting the pen off the paper, and you will be asked to sign your name. The waviness of the spiral and the size and waviness of the signature will tell your doctor whether your tremor is more likely due to ET, Parkinson's disease, or some other condition. It also gives your doctor an idea of the severity of your tremor.

Your doctor will rate your tremor on a scale from 0 to 4. A "0" means no tremor at all, "1" is a mild tremor, "2" is moderate, "3" is moderately severe, and "4" is severe. People with a "3" or "4" on the tremor scale always will be given treatment recommendations. A "2" on the tremor scale can still be very disabling for some people and may need treatment as well. Insurance companies often look carefully at these rating scales when deciding whether to cover the cost of certain treatments, like deep brain stimulation (DBS), gamma knife, or focused ultrasound. Please see the chapter on surgical treatments for more information about these. Most of the time, you need a tremor of grade "3" or "4" to qualify for those treatments, although there can be exceptions.

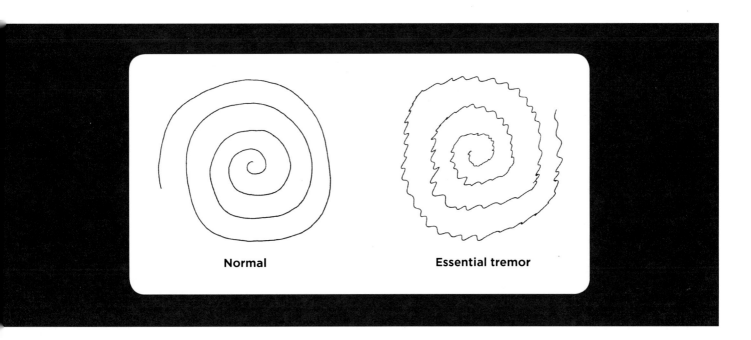

Normal   **Essential tremor**

VIDEOTAPING

Some doctors will want to videotape parts of your exam, especially those parts that show your tremor. This usually happens if you are being considered for surgery, gamma knife, or focused ultrasound treatment. Many neurologists, especially in large medical centers, will recommend whether or not you should have surgery based on conferences with other neurologists, neuro-surgeons, psychologists, and other doctors who take care of you. In these conferences, video recordings of patients' tremors are often shown so that doctors who have not seen you in person can get an idea of how bad your tremor is. This helps everyone make the best recommendations for you. Videotaping can also be helpful if you decide to have surgery or other treatments. Often, you will be videotaped again a few months after surgery so your doctor can compare before and after videos to see how much better you have gotten. My patients are often amazed at how much certain treatments have helped when they see the differences between these videos!

Discussion about what may be causing your problem

While your doctor is asking you about your medical history and examining you, he or she is using all of this information to figure out what is causing you to shake. Sometimes the information your doctor gets during this visit is enough to be able to figure out the problem. However, sometimes you will need more tests, such as blood tests or certain types of x-rays, to help him or her figure out your "diagnosis," or what is causing your tremor. In either case, your doctor will spend a few minutes talking to you (and any family members who have come with you, if you are comfortable with them being there) about the things that could be causing your tremor. Your doctor will also talk to you about what other tests to get, or specialists to see, to help him or her decide what your diagnosis is.

This is a good time to ask questions about anything you do not understand. Also, ask your doctor about anything else that has been bothering you about your health, even if you think those issues have nothing to do with your tremor. Your doctor is there to help you with your medical concerns. If he or she does not know the answer, your doctor will know which other kind of doctor you should see in order to find out the answers. Some people find it helpful to bring in a list of questions to ask and then go through that list with their doctor. One other bit of advice I can give you is this: once your doctor has finished telling you his or her thoughts and recommendations, it is a great idea to use your own words to repeat back what the doctor has just said. This may seem silly at first. But if you think about it, this will make sure that you really understand everything, and your doctor will be able to clear up any misunderstandings you have.

In the past few years, I have started asking my patients to tell me what they understood I have just said to them. I have been amazed at the number of times that this part of the discussion has made a difference in helping patients understand what I say. Sometimes we doctors give so much information at once that it can be overwhelming. Then our patients understandably miss the most important things we have said! Finally, if your doctor does not give you a "printout" at the end of your visit with next steps and instructions, then you may want to write down in a notebook a list things you need to do next, such as get blood drawn or see a different doctor.

During your discussion with your doctor:

- *Listen carefully*
- *Ask questions about what your doctor says*
- *Ask other questions you have about your health*
- *Repeat back to your doctor, in your own words, what he or she has told you*
- *Write down the instructions your doctor gives you*

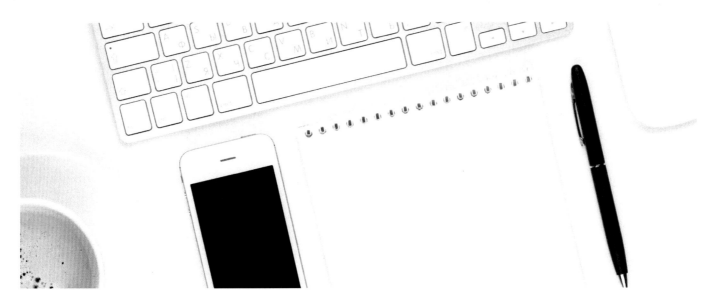

Lab studies

There are blood tests that can help your doctor figure out why you are shaking. For example, if the sugar levels in your blood are not normal, or if your thyroid is not working properly, this may cause you to shake. (Often these would cause shaking through your whole body rather than in just one arm or leg.) These blood tests involve having blood drawn out of your arm and often can be done the same day as your appointment. Your doctor will either schedule a follow-up visit or call you to discuss the results. Be sure to ask your doctor how you will find out the results and set a reminder to call your doctor in a week if you have not heard from the office.

X-ray studies

Certain x-ray studies, such as CT or MRI scans, can also give your doctor information about the cause of your tremor. These usually have to be scheduled and some may require your doctor to send a letter to your insurance company so they will pay for the scan. So, it is likely you will not be able to have these tests the same day as your doctor's visit. As with lab tests, your doctor will either schedule a follow-up visit or call you to discuss the results. Call your doctor to get the results a week after your scan or scans if you have not heard from him or her.

Referrals to other medical professionals

Your doctor may suggest that you see other medical professionals to help either figure out your diagnosis or give you more options for treatment. These recommendations are called "referrals" and may include: another neurologist who has more expertise treating people with tremors; an occupational therapist who can help you learn ways to work around your tremors and do the things you want to do; a psychologist who can help you manage stress and other problems like depression or anxiety; or a neurosurgeon who can talk to you about possible surgeries to help your tremor. Please see the next chapter for an explanation of each of these types of medical providers and what to expect during those visits.

Follow-up visits

Often your neurologist will want to see you again to discuss test results or to follow-up on recommendations your referrals gave you. Your doctor may decide to treat you him or herself or "transfer your care" to another doctor. A transfer of care usually happens if your doctor is not a specialist in treating people who have movement disorders like essential tremor, and it means the new doctor will make recommendations to you on the treatment of your tremors from that point on. If you have a new problem, you then can go back to see your general practitioner or general neurologist. Be sure to ask your doctor before the end of your visit whether he or she will see you for more appointments, follow up with you by phone, or transfer your care to another doctor.

Where to go for your appointment

Depending on what type of doctor you see and where you have your appointment, your experience at the doctor may be a little different. The next chapter describes the experiences you may have when you see different types of doctors. You also will have a choice about whether to see a doctor who works independently or in an office with other doctors in either a "private practice" or an "academic medical center." Academic medical centers often can offer multiple appointments with different kinds of medical providers on the same day or within a few days of one another. Some patients with tremor prefer this. Also, academic medical centers often treat patients who have complicated medical problems that some private practice doctors do not have experience treating.

In any case, when you see a doctor who works independently, it is important to ask how much he or she interacts with other specialists who work with patients with tremor. Personally, I am biased towards the "team-based approach" for patients with tremor. This approach does not necessarily mean that your doctor has to be part of a big hospital system—it means that your doctor should have frequent referrals back and forth with the other doctors who will be helping with your care. This will help ensure that you have the most complete treatment available.

CHAPTER SUMMARY

At your doctor's appointment, you will answer questions, have a medical exam, talk to your doctor about possible causes of your tremor, and discuss your next steps. The parts of your visit include:

- Medical history
  - Information about when you shake, what shakes, when the shaking first started
  - Questions about your other medical problems
  - Screening questions about how shaking affects your life

- Physical exam
  - Examination of your memory and knowledge
  - Examination of the nerves in your brain, arms, and legs
  - A "tremor exam"

- Discussion and recommendations
  - Blood tests
  - X-rays: CT scans, MRI scans
  - Referrals to other medical providers

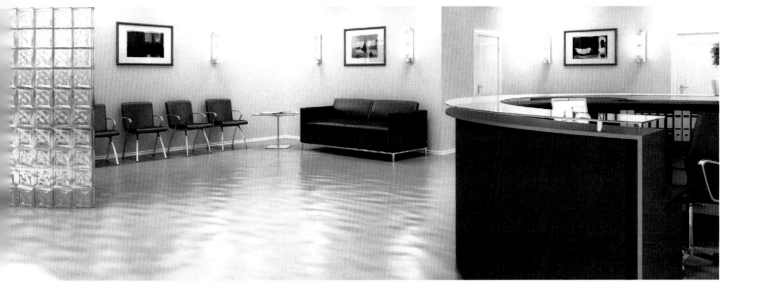

MEDICAL PROVIDERS AND MEDICINES

In this chapter, you will learn about the different kinds of medical providers who evaluate and treat people who have tremors. The term "medical provider" includes doctors and other trained professionals who evaluate and treat you for various conditions. Also in this chapter is a description of medicines that you may be offered to help decrease your tremor.

FAMILY MEDICINE AND INTERNAL MEDICINE

Family medicine and internal medicine doctors see both healthy people and people with all kinds of medical problems. Some people call these doctors "GPs," which stands for "general practitioners," because they treat so many different problems. Sometimes, a GP will have a good idea about the cause of your tremor and may order medicines for you. If these medicines are working, the GP may not refer you to a neurologist. It is a good idea to see a neurologist, or a movement disorder neurologist if you have tremors, even if your GP is confident treating your condition. Neurologists have more in-depth training in the treatment of tremors and are often aware much sooner about new medicines and treatments that could help you with your tremors. You can ask your family medicine doctor or internal medicine doctor for a referral to a neurologist, or to a movement disorder neurologist if you have tremor.

NEUROLOGY AND MOVEMENT DISORDER NEUROLOGY

A **neurologist** is a doctor who specializes in examining and treating people who have problems with their brains, spinal cords, or nerves. This doctor likely will be able to tell you what condition you have that is causing you to shake and may order some of the tests described in the last chapter in order to figure this out. If this neurologist is not sure what is causing you to shake, he or she will send you to a movement disorder neurologist (see below), who may order more tests. A general neurologist sometimes will order medicines for you to take to help reduce your tremors, if he or she is fairly certain about your diagnosis. The neurologist will also refer you to other medical providers, described in this section, who will help you in other ways.

A **movement disorder neurologist** is a doctor who specializes in treating people with conditions that affect their ability to move their bodies normally, such as essential tremor (ET), Parkinson's disease, and others. Because this doctor specializes in movement disorders, he or she will almost always be able to tell you what is causing your tremor. Sometimes this doctor will order tests, described in the last chapter, in order to figure out your diagnosis. Like a general neurologist, a movement disorder neurologist may order medicines in the form of pills for you. He or she may also order medicines that have to be "injected" or given as a "shot." A movement disorder neurologist may refer you to the other providers described in this section, if he or she thinks you need more treatment.

What to expect

When you see a general or movement disorder neurologist, you can expect to have the evaluation that is described in the previous chapter.

MEDICINES

As mentioned above, there are medicines that can help reduce tremors in some people. Most of these are pills that you take by mouth. There is another medicine that can also help tremors in some people, which needs to be given by injection in order to work. This is called a "Botox" treatment.

Pills

There are two common types of medicines that are given to control tremors caused by ET. These are "beta blockers" and medicines that were originally made to stop shaking in people who have seizures. Usually, your doctor will order one of the two types of medicines to start with. You may also take both at the same time if one is not working. There are other medicines that can sometimes be given to decrease your tremors; however, they usually do not work as well as these first two types of medicines. Because of this, usually you will only take these other medicines in addition to one of the first two, or if neither of the first two medicines work.

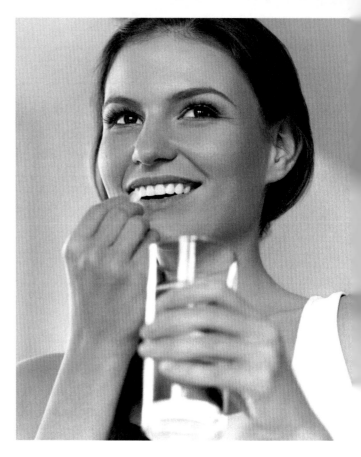

BETA BLOCKERS (PROPRANOLOL, METOPROLOL, AND OTHERS)

What they are

Beta blockers are one of the most common types of medicine given to reduce tremors. They are a group of medicines often "prescribed," or given, to lower blood pressure or treat heart problems after a heart attack. Beta blockers have been shown to cut the amount of hand and arm tremors in half in about 50% of people with ET.[1] They may help with voice tremors as well.[2] The most commonly prescribed beta blocker is propranolol, which has several brand names, the most common of which is Inderal.

Who can take them

Many people can take beta blockers, with a few important exceptions. You cannot take beta blockers if you have breathing conditions like asthma, emphysema, or chronic bronchitis, or if you have certain problems with your heart rate (the number of times per minute your heart beats).[3] For example, if your heart rate is less than 50 beats per minute, it may not be safe to take a beta blocker. Propranolol may be safe to take when you are pregnant or breast-feeding. Be sure to tell a doctor who is ordering beta blockers for you about other medical problems you have and other medicines you are taking.

It is also a good idea to talk to your pharmacist about this medicine when you pick up your prescription. Most pharmacists will offer a free consultation to tell you how to take your medicine and will go over the side effects it can have. Also, if you look up your medicine on Drugs.com, there is a section called "Drug Interactions." There, you can type in your other medicine and see if taking it together with your beta blocker will cause problems. If you take a lot of other medicines, you should check the interactions of the beta blocker with each of your other medicines.

How to take them

In most cases, you will take propranolol twice a day, at the same times every day. Usually your doctor will start you off on a low dose, around 40 mg taken twice a day.[4] The maximum dose of propranolol for ET is 160 mg taken twice a day. You should try to take your two daily doses twelve hours apart, such as 7 am and 7 pm every day. You do not have to take this medication with food, but you can if you want to.

Side effects

The most common side effects from beta blockers are tiredness, low heart rate, dizziness, depression, and low sex drive.[5] Up to half of the people who take beta blockers have some side effects. Switching to a different beta blocker may help to decrease your side effects, so talk to your doctor if they are bothering you.

Cost and insurance

Propranolol may cost about $50 a month if you are on the common dose of 60 mg twice a day.[6] Most insurance companies will cover the cost of beta blockers for the treatment of ET. You should check with your insurance company to see if it covers this medicine. If your insurance company refuses to cover the cost of your treatment at first, your doctor can always write a "letter of appeal." This is not a guarantee that the company will agree to pay for the treatment, but it does increase the chances that it will.

PRIMIDONE (MYSOLINE)

What it is

Primidone, or Mysoline, is the other very common medicine given to control tremors. This medicine is often given to stop seizures. Like beta blockers, primidone has been shown to cut tremors in half in about 50% of people with ET.[7] It also may help decrease voice tremors.[8]

Who can take it

Most people can take primidone. If you cannot take beta blockers for any reason, your doctor will probably order primidone for you instead. You cannot take primidone if you are pregnant or breastfeeding, because it can cause serious birth defects.[9] Be sure to talk to your doctor and pharmacist about other medical problems you have and other medicines you are taking to be sure that primidone is safe for you to take.

How to take it

You will take primidone once a day in the beginning and will take it up to three times a day after a few weeks. The reason the dose gradually goes up is to make it less likely that you will have side effects and to figure out what dose you need to control your tremor. Usually you will start taking 50 mg of primidone once at night and increase your dose a little bit every week, up to a maximum dose of 100 mg taken three times a day. You may be given higher doses; however, more than 300 mg of primidone per day may not help your tremors and may give you more side effects.[10] You can take primidone with or without food and, as with propranolol, you should take it at the same time every day.

Side effects

The main side effects are sleepiness, dizziness, confusion, and upset stomach.[5] Up to half the people who take primidone have side effects that bother them enough to stop taking this medicine.

Cost and insurance

Primidone may cost around $45 a month, if you are taking 300 mg per day.[11] As with propranolol, most insurance companies will cover the cost of this medicine for ET. You should check with your insurance company to see whether they cover this medicine.

Other pills

Other medicines that have been used to control ET include the following:

- *Gabapentin (Neurontin)*
- *Alprazolam (Xanax)*
- *Topiramate (Topamax)*

These medicines decrease tremors by 20% to 30% and may cause major side effects, including severe sleepiness. There are even more medicines that may help some people with tremors. If none of the medicines described in this book are helping to control your tremors, talk to your doctor to see what other options are available.

Botox

Botulinum neurotoxin, or Botox, is a medicine that is injected into your muscles by your doctor. It is generally used to treat voice tremor, by an injection into the vocal cords in your throat. Botox usually will start to work as soon as two days after the injection, and it can control your tremor for around six weeks. The major side effects from Botox injections include difficulty swallowing and a voice that is softer or raspier than normal.[12] Those side effects usually go away when the Botox wears off and your voice tremor comes back. Botox also has been tried for treatment of hand and head tremors and can help somewhat in these cases. However, it causes significant muscle weakness in many people, making Botox an undesirable treatment for any tremors other than voice tremors.[13]

NEUROSURGERY

A neurosurgeon is a doctor who specializes in using surgery to treat people who have problems with their brains, spinal cords, or nerves. Just because you see a neurosurgeon as a patient in his or her office does NOT mean you will be having surgery! Often a visit to a neurosurgeon is only to tell you what kinds of surgery may be able to help your tremor and/or to evaluate whether you are healthy enough to have surgery. A neurosurgeon may recommend that you have one of the surgeries described in the next chapter or that you have no surgery at all. As a patient, you always have the right to decide NOT to have medical or surgical treatment. As a practicing neurosurgeon, I probably only tell about half of the patients I see to have surgery.

Things a neurosurgeon can do for you:

- Tell you about the different surgeries that can help your tremor
- Tell you if you are healthy enough for surgery
- Do your surgeries

WHAT TO EXPECT

When you see a neurosurgeon, you can expect to have an evaluation, which is described in the next chapter.

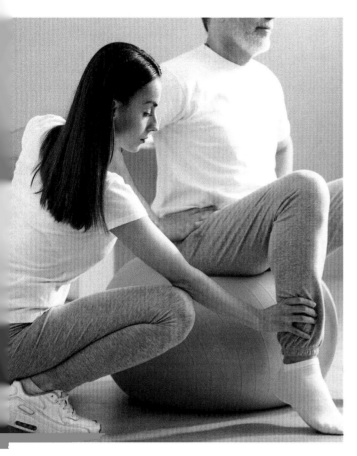

OCCUPATIONAL THERAPY

Occupational therapists, or OTs, help people live full lives by teaching them ways to keep from getting hurt or helping them do the things they want to do when they have an injury, disease, or sickness.[14] Often occupational therapists will help people with tremors learn ways to eat and drink without spilling, get dressed more easily, write more legibly, and enjoy their hobbies again.

Things an OT can help you do more easily:

- *Learn to eat soup and peas*
- *Drink without spilling*
- *Write your name so people can read it*
- *Use a computer keyboard or mouse more easily*

To do these things, an occupational therapist may teach you exercises to strengthen muscles and increase coordination, slightly different ways to do your activities, and how to use "assistive devices" (tools designed to help people overcome tremor).

What to expect

The first time you see an occupational therapist, you can expect him or her to spend a lot of time asking you questions about ways your tremors affect your life. Your OT will ask how your tremors affect your "activities of daily living," or ADLs. These are the things you need to do to live daily, like eat and drink, get dressed, and take a shower or bath. Your OT will also ask you how your tremors affect your job (if you are working) and your ability to do your hobbies. Make sure to mention if you have stopped going out in public, such as to restaurants or other places, because you are embarrassed about your tremor. The more information your OT has about what is bothering you, the better he or she will be able to give you advice and make a specific plan to help you.

Your OT will do a physical exam and may ask you to do things like write, pretend to drink from a cup, and many of the other things that you also did during your appointment with the neurologist. This is not meant to embarrass you. Your OT needs to see firsthand which activities give you the most trouble so that he or she can help you. It is very difficult for an OT to read another doctor's office notes and make a plan for you without seeing your tremors in person.

Your OT will then develop a "treatment plan" for you. In the sections below, I explain in more detail some of the more common ways an OT may help you with your tremor. You may start with your treatment plan on the first visit, or the first visit may just be an evaluation. Most likely, you will be asked to come back every week or so to continue with your therapy.

Cost and insurance

In general, most occupational therapy visits will be paid for by your insurance company, although you will need a "prescription" from your neurologist or internal medicine/family medicine doctor. Often your insurance company will approve a certain number of times you can see an OT. Your OT should be able to teach you exercises, show you new ways to do your daily activities, and let you test out assistive devices in just a few visits.

COMMON TECHNIQUES AN OT WILL USE TO HELP WITH YOUR TREMOR

These techniques are described in much more detail in Section 2 of this book. Below, I describe the ways an OT will help you use these techniques. Most of them are designed for you to eventually be able to use on your own.

Exercises

Strengthening your muscles will make your arms and legs much less likely to shake. Most of the exercises your OT teaches you will make your hands, arms, and fingers stronger. Your OT may also teach you ways to make your mid-section, or "core," stronger. When you use your abdominal muscles to stabilize your body, your arms and legs do not have to do as much work, and this makes you shake less. Your OT will be able to pick out the best exercises for you to help you reach your goals. For example, if your tremor bothers you most when you are trying to knit, your OT will give you more exercises for your hands, wrists, and fingers; if you want to improve your woodworking ability, your OT will give you more exercises for your arms and core.

Your OT will show you how to do the exercises and then watch you do them, to make sure you get the most benefit from your exercises by doing them safely and correctly. If you have follow-up visits with your OT, he or she will give you instructions on how often to do your exercises and then watch you do them again when you come back. This is helpful for many reasons. First, your OT can make sure you are still doing the exercises in a safe and effective way. Second, your OT will get information on whether the exercises have made it easier for you to do the things you want to do. Your OT will suggest new exercises or change your exercises a little bit if you are not getting the results you wanted.

Assistive Tools

Your OT should have many assistive tools in his or her office that you can try out. This is helpful for many reasons. Some tools, such as weighted spoons and forks, have many companies that make them and may all be slightly different. By testing them out with your OT, you will know which ones to buy and not have to deal with returning items that are not working well. Also, if you try out one set of weighted utensils on your own, and they do not work, then you may think that all weighted utensils are worthless. You could be missing out on something that would really help you, if you only knew which model was best for you!

Further, some of the products can be expensive, especially those that have electronic components or computer software, such as Liftware Steady™ and computer mice. Items with computer and phone software can also require some getting used to and could get frustrating if you tried them out on your own. Your OT can help you set up and learn to use these items so you get the most out of them, and you will be able see if they help you enough to make it worth the money. This also helps you avoid having to return items, although most of the more expensive ones give you a money-back guarantee.

Different ways to do everyday tasks

Your OT can help you learn new ways to do the things you want to do every day without having to buy any equipment. I have described many of these techniques in Section 2 of this book. Not everyone needs all of these techniques, and your OT may help you change some of them a little bit to fit your specific situation. For example, if you have tremors but also a lot of stiffness in your arms, your OT can suggest ways to adjust common tremor techniques so you can still use them.

Therapies

There are a few therapies that your OT may try to see if they help your tremor. The only one that has been proven to slow down ET is hand and arm cooling. Others, such as vibration therapy and bright light therapy, have been shown to slow down tremors in Parkinson's disease.[15,16] However, we do not really understand how those work to slow down tremor, so it is not known whether they will help slow down shaking that is caused by ET.

Hand and arm cooling

Cooling hands and arms to around 59 degrees Fahrenheit (15 degrees Celsius) for five minutes at a time, up to 30 minutes total, can reduce tremor in some people for a few hours.[17] Often, this is done by placing your hands in cool water.[18,19] It is important that you DO NOT try to do this yourself! You need to be watched by a medical professional, such as an OT, to make sure you are not having any serious side effects from this treatment. Cooling a hand or arm for too long can slow down the blood that is getting to your hand. In certain cases, you could possibly lose a finger if you tried to do this yourself!

PSYCHOLOGY

As described in the first section of this book, it is common for people with tremors to have some problems with depression (sadness lasting more than two weeks), anxiety (nervousness), and cognitive problems, such as difficulty planning and thinking through problems. Up to half of all people who have tremors are depressed, and one-third have anxiety. For some people, their anxiety or nervousness is so bad that they don't even want to leave the house. Recently, researchers have discovered that people who have a lot of anxiety also have worse tremors.[20] They do not know whether anxiety makes tremors worse, or whether tremors make anxiety worse. Either way, there is help for people with tremors who have depression, anxiety, or cognitive problems.

A psychologist is a medical professional who helps people with issues such as depression, anxiety, and stress by teaching them ways to cope with these problems. A psychologist has a degree called a PhD, as opposed to the MD or DO degree that your medical doctor, neurologist, and neurosurgeon have. Some can order medicines, depending on the state where they have their license and the type of training they have, while others may recommend medicines that your general medical doctor can order. There are certain psychologists who have special training in working with people who have tremors and other neurological problems. They are known as "neuropsychologists." These doctors can also help figure out if you have any cognitive problems.

A psychologist can help with the following:

- *Tell you if you are depressed, anxious, or have other psychological conditions*
- *Teach you ways to be less stressed, less nervous, and less sad*
- *Recommend or order medicines to help with depression, anxiety or stress*
- *A neuropsychologist can tell you if you have cognitive problems*

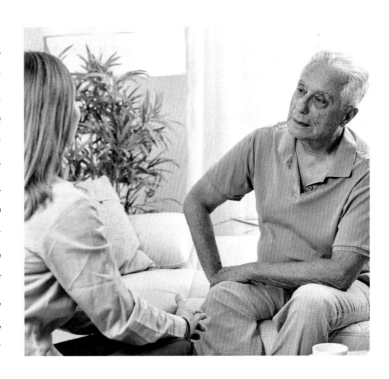

Your first appointment with a psychologist will probably take about an hour to an hour and a half. A lot of time will be spent filling out paperwork and answering questions about yourself, your past, and what is bothering you most right now. When you see the psychologist, he or she will want to know about your medical problems. Take the time to explain how your tremors are making you feel and what kinds of things you cannot do because of your tremors. All of this is confidential, so you can feel free to tell your psychologist everything that is bothering you, without worrying that he or she will tell anyone else. Remember that even if you are going to a psychologist to talk about ways your tremor affects your life, you can use your time to talk about any problems that are bothering you! As with the other medical professionals, the more information you give your psychologist, the more he or she will be able to help you.

Your later visits with the psychologist will focus more on figuring out why you feel the way you feel and ways you can change your feelings to become happier and more relaxed. Usually these appointments last about an hour. You may see your psychologist once a week, twice a month, or once a month, depending on what you discuss at the first appointment and what your doctor recommends. Most people with tremor will see a psychologist for a few months to a year, while others may continue to see one for several years. This is a very personalized treatment, and you will get the most help by following the advice of your doctor.

If you see a neuropsychologist rather than a general psychologist, you will likely have only one visit, and it will be very different from what I described above. A neuropsychologist will give you many different "tests" to determine your ability to think through and solve problems. He or she will also test your memory. These tests can take between two and three hours, in addition to the hour or so spent talking to you about your past and current problems. So eat a good meal before going to this visit! If you are considering having surgery to treat your tremors, you should see a neuropsychologist at least once before your surgery. You also will probably have a follow-up appointment with a neuropsychologist a few months after your surgery.

NOTE: In Section 2 of this book, I describe many ways you can work to lower your own stress and improve your cognitive function. These are not meant to replace professional help from a psychologist—they are meant to be done in addition to this treatment.

Cost and insurance

First visits to a psychologist usually cost between $150 to $300. Follow-up visits usually cost between $75 and $150. A neuropsychologist visit likely will cost over $1000. Most insurance companies will cover the cost of a few visits with a psychologist and one or two visits with a neuropsychologist. You should contact your insurance company to find out how many visits they will cover. Some insurance companies have a "lifetime" limit on psychologist's visits, so if you have seen a psychologist in the past for other reasons and still have the same insurance, you may have to pay for your visits. If you have to pay for visits yourself, you often can find a free clinic or a discounted appointments through your local university if you agree to see a student who is almost finished training.[21]

Medical provider	How they can help
Family or internal medicine / GP	Give medicines Refer you to a specialist
Neurologist	Tell you what kind of tremor you have Give medicines
Movement disorder neurologist	Tell you what kind of tremor you have Give medicines Give botox
Neurosurgeon	Tell you about surgery choices Do your surgery
Occupational therapist	Teach you to eat and drink without spilling Teach you how to communicate more easily
Psychologist	Teach you how to be happier and calmer
Neuropsychologist	Tell you if you have cognitive problems

REFERENCES

1. Hedera P, Cibulčík F, Davis TL. Pharmacotherapy of essential tremor. *J Cent Nerv Syst Dis*. 2013;5:43–55.

2. Justicz N, Hapner ER, Josephs JS, Boone BC, Jinnah HA, Johns MM. Comparative effectiveness of propranolol and botulinum for the treatment of essential voice tremor. Laryngoscope. 2016;126(1):113-7.

3. Drugs.com. Contraindications. https://www.drugs.com/pro/propranolol.html.

4. Drugs.com. Usual Adult Dose for Benign Essential Tremor. https://www.drugs.com/dosage/propranolol.html#Usual_Adult_Dose_for_Benign_Essential_Tremor.

5. Gironell A, Kulisevsky J. Diagnosis and management of essential tremor and dystonic tremor. *Ther Adv Neurol Disord*. 2009;2(4):215–222.

6. Drugs.com. Propranolol Prices, Coupons, and Patient Assistance Programs. https://www.drugs.com/price-guide/propranolol.

7. Rajput AH, Rajput A. Medical treatment of essential tremor. *J Cent Nerv Syst Dis*. 2014;6:29–39.

8. Nida A, Alston J, Schweinfurth J. Primidone therapy for essential vocal tremor. *JAMA Otolaryngol Head Neck Surg*. 2016;142(2):117-21.

9. Drugs.com Primidone Pregnancy Warnings. https://www.drugs.com/pregnancy/primidone.html.

10. Hedera P, Cibulcik F, and Davis TL. Pharmacotherapy of Essential Tremor. *J Cent Nerv Syst Dis*. 2013;5:43–55.

11. Drugs.com. Primidone Prices, Coupons, and Patient Assistance Programs. https://www.drugs.com/price-guide/primidone.

12. Adler CH, Bansberg SF, Hentz JG, et al. Botulinum Toxin Type A for Treating Voice Tremor. *Arch Neurol*. 2004;61(9):1416-1420.

13. Brin MF, Lyons KE, Doucette J, et al. A randomized, double masked, controlled trial of botulinum toxin type A in essential hand tremor. *Neurology*. 2001;56(11):1523-8.

14. International Essential Tremor Foundation. An Occupational Therapy Perspective. https://www.essentialtremor.org/coping/coping-with-et-articles/an-occupational-therapy-perspective/.

15. Paus S, Schmitz-Hübsch T, Wüllner U, Vogel A, Klockgether T, Abele M. Bright light therapy in Parkinson's disease: a pilot study. *Mov Disord*. 2007;22(10):1495-8.

16. King LK, Almeida QJ, Ahonen H. Short-term effects of vibration therapy on motor impairments in Parkinson's disease. *NeuroRehabilitation*. 2009;25(4):297-306.

17. Tremor Action Network. Occupational Therapies for Essential Tremor. http://tremoraction.org/2016/10/occupational-therapies-for-essential-tremor.

18. Lakie M, Walsh EG, Arblaster LA, Villagra F, Roberts RC. Limb temperature and human tremors. *J Neurol Neurosurg Psychiatry*. 1994;57(1):35-42.

19. Cooper C, Evidente VG, Hentz JG, Adler CH, Caviness JN, Gwinn-Hardy K. The effect of temperature on hand function in patients with tremor. *J Hand Ther*. 2000;13(4):276-88.

20. Smeltere L, Kuzņecovs V, Erts R. Depression and social phobia in essential tremor and Parkinson's disease. *Brain Behav*. 2017;7(9):e00781.

21. Bergen A. How to Find Affordable Therapy or Counseling. Money under 30. https://www.moneyunder30.com/affordable-therapy.

SURGICAL TREATMENT

You may not realize it, but there are surgeries that can help tremors due to essential tremor (ET) or Parkinson's disease. The idea of surgery may sound a little frightening at first. But if you understand what happens during the surgery and learn how much surgery can help you, you might feel more comfortable with the idea of it. Not everyone needs surgery. Many people are able to use a combination of self-care treatments and medicines to control their tremors enough that they can do most of the things they want to do. As I describe each type of surgical procedure below, I will tell you who could be helped by the surgery and who should probably not have the surgery. I will also tell you what to expect during each procedure. Finally, I will share with you how you can expect your symptoms to change if you choose to have the surgery.

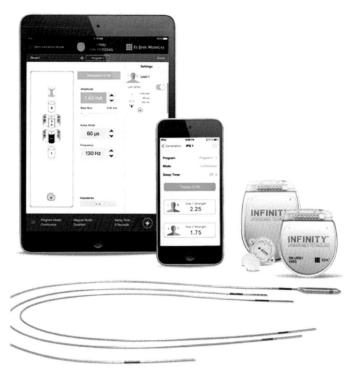

Photo credit: St. Jude Medical Infinity™ DBS system by Abbott

DEEP BRAIN STIMULATION

What it is

Deep Brain Stimulation, or "DBS," is a surgery that involves placing tiny wires deep inside the brain. These wires are called "electrodes," and have metal contacts on the ends of them. Pulses of electricity are sent through these metal contacts to an area of the brain that controls tremors. This area of the brain is called the "thalamus," and specifically an area in the thalamus known as the "Vim" (pronounced "vee - eye - em"). The electrical pulses are controlled by a small device that is placed in the chest (sometimes called a brain "pacemaker") and connected to the electrodes in the brain by a wire. All the pieces of the DBS system are placed underneath the skin, so you won't have any wires hanging out of your body.

One of the greatest benefits of DBS over treatments like Gamma Knife or focused ultrasound (see below) is that DBS can be adjusted or removed at any time. You can remove it if you are having trouble with the system or if a cure for tremors is found that requires you to take out your system. You can also adjust your DBS system, which is important, since tremors often get worse over time. The ability to "turn up" the system when tremors get worse means this treatment can work for many, many years. DBS as a treatment for tremor was first discovered by Dr. Alim-Louis Benabid, one of my mentors in neurosurgery, with whom I had the privilege of working closely in France between 2011 and 2012. Dr. Benabid discovered this treatment for tremors due to ET and Parkinson's disease in 1987,[1] and DBS has been approved for this use since 1997.[2]

There are many factors that can impact whether or not surgery is a good solution for your tremor. These include the severity of your tremor, your overall physical and mental health, and the medicines you may be taking.

TREMOR SEVERITY

DBS is considered for people whose tremor greatly affects their lives. This includes people who have a lot of trouble eating, buttoning buttons, zipping zippers, writing, typing on a keyboard, or safely doing their jobs at work. It also includes people who cannot do the hobbies they love and enjoy, such as knitting, playing golf, woodworking, playing an instrument, or painting, because of their tremor. As I mentioned earlier in the book, some people only have tremors when doing very specific activities. If you only have tremors when you play violin, for example, and you play second string for your orchestra, this is enough reason to be considered for DBS surgery. Even if your day-to-day activities are not limited by your tremor, sometimes the social challenges you have when others see you shaking in public are enough to consider surgery. Importantly, you must not be able to control your tremor through self-help and medicines in order to be considered for DBS surgery. If you can control your tremor using other methods, it does not make any sense to take the risks that come with surgery.

Overall physical health and medicines you take

There is no specific age limit for DBS surgery; however, you need to be medically and psychologically healthy enough to have surgery. If you have had a heart attack or even bypass surgery a few years ago, but your cardiologist thinks you are now healthy enough for surgery, then you may still be able to get DBS. But if you had a heart attack a few months ago, your doctors will probably tell you to wait a year or so before having the surgery. People who have had heart surgery, stents, or other procedures sometimes have to take medicine that thins the blood. They often wonder if they can still have brain surgery. The answer is: Sometimes.

Most people who are taking blood thinners can safely stop taking them for a short period—two to three weeks—around the time of surgery. If the doctor who put you on the blood thinner says this is safe, then yes, you can still have DBS. It is very important that patients stop taking most blood thinners about 7 to 10 days before surgery and wait to restart the medicines until a few days after surgery. This is because there is a risk of bleeding inside the brain with DBS or any other brain surgery. This risk is much higher if you take medicines that thin the blood. Some people don't realize that aspirin and ibuprofen are also blood thinners and cannot be taken within a week or so of surgery. Some vitamins, such as Vitamin E, and some medicines, such as carbamazepine, also thin the blood.[3]

If you bleed or bruise very easily, you should have your doctor do a full check-up, including blood tests and other procedures, to be sure your do not have hemophilia or another issue that keeps your blood from clotting normally. People with bleeding disorders cannot safely have DBS surgery. You also may have to wait to have DBS if you have an infection. Even a cold, flu, or bladder infection can delay a surgery. If you have severe lung problems, like COPD (chronic obstructive pulmonary disorder), that are not well controlled with medicines, you also may not be able to have DBS. There can be problems with going to sleep for and waking up from surgery with this condition. Overall, any condition you have for which your primary care doctor says surgery is not safe would keep you from having DBS surgery.

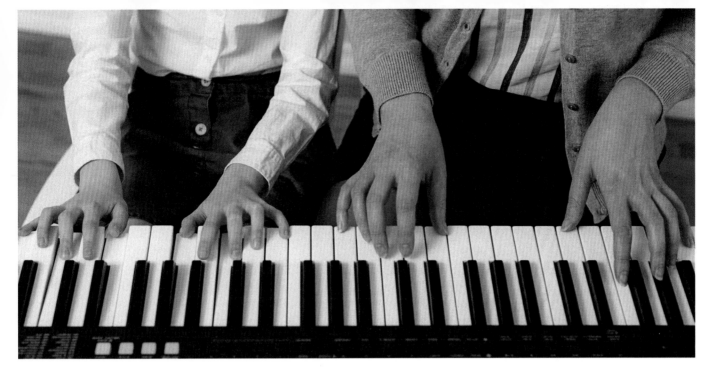

Mental health and dementia

If you have chronic depression or anxiety (a common issue for people with tremors), but it is under control with counseling and/or medication, then you would still be a good candidate for surgery. However, if you had a suicide attempt a few months ago, your doctors will probably have you wait a few more months to be sure your mental state is stable before considering surgery. If you have severe memory loss or dementia, you also would not be a good candidate for DBS. People with dementia have difficulty with DBS for a few reasons. They may have trouble during the "awake" part of the surgery, when they need to answer the doctor's questions. They also may have trouble remembering to come to follow-up appointments and following instructions on taking care of themselves after surgery.

Good candidate	Poor candidate
Severe tremors limiting lifestyle	Mild tremor not affecting lifestyle
Tremor not controlled with medicines	Tremor well controlled with medicines
Recovered from heart attack over 1 year ago	Recent heart attack
Safely can stop blood thinners for 2-3 weeks	Cannot stop taking blood thinning medicines
	Current infection
	Severe lung problems
	Depression got worse/recent suicide attempt
	Severe uncontrolled anxiety
	Dementia

Evaluation

First of all, expect it to take some time to get an evaluation, or exam to see if you are a good candidate, for DBS. Most neurosurgeons will require you to see a movement disorder neurologist before considering surgery. You may be videotaped during this examination in order to record the severity of your tremor. You probably will also need an evaluation by a neuropsychologist to figure out if you have dementia or an untreated condition like depression or anxiety.

You will need a special x-ray of your brain called an MRI, or magnetic resonance image. This involves lying flat on a narrow table, having a small "coil," which looks somewhat like a cage, placed over your head, and then being put into a tunnel-like machine. You will hear loud banging sounds during the scan, and during certain times you will be asked to hold your breath. Some MRIs have mirrors placed so you can see outside the scanner. This helps people feel less "claustrophobic," or scared of being in a closed space. If you cannot have an MRI of the brain—due to having certain types of metal in in your body—you may have a CT, or computerized tomography, scan instead.

Then, you will be evaluated for DBS surgery by a neurosurgeon. The neurosurgeon will describe the way he or she does the surgery, discuss the risks, and give you instructions about surgery. Sometimes, after this evaluation, you may be asked to see your primary care doctor to figure out if you are healthy enough for surgery, or you may be asked to see a specialist if your neurosurgeon is concerned about a specific condition. Some doctors then meet with the entire team who has evaluated you before making a decision about surgery. These team meetings allow each of your doctors to discuss opinions and concerns about you as a candidate for surgery. In some larger medical centers, other doctors of the same specialties may be involved in the discussion as well.

If the doctors decide that you are a good candidate for surgery, you will be called and offered the procedure. If you decide to go ahead with the surgery, then the neurosurgeon's office will send paperwork to your insurance company to find out if your insurance plan will cover the procedure. This can be a frustrating time for people waiting to have surgery. Most insurance companies will cover DBS. However, many of them need specific information in a doctor's note in order to approve the surgery, and sometimes the doctor's office will have to call the insurance company to get the surgery approved.

If you are being evaluated at a large academic medical center, you can expect it to take 6-8 months from your first evaluation to your actual surgery. About a week or so prior to your actual surgery date, you will need to have blood drawn, x-rays of your chest, and possibly another MRI or CT scan of your brain. If anything in these tests comes back abnormal, your surgery could be delayed—though this is very rarely the case.

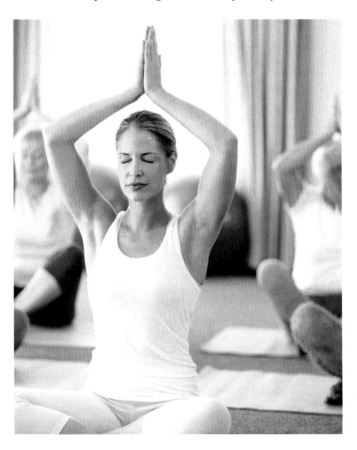

Surgery

What will happen during your surgery can vary a lot depending on the preferences of your surgeon. There are many ways that DBS surgery can be performed. Some of these require you to be awake during surgery, and others require the use of an MRI machine. Some surgeons use a metal frame that is attached to your skull, while others use a system that does not need a frame. There are two parts to every DBS surgery. The first part involves a brain surgery to place one or two electrodes in the brain. The second part involves connecting the brain electrodes to a "pacemaker" that is placed in your chest below your collarbone. Below is a description of the different ways the first part of the DBS surgery can be done and what to expect with each type of procedure. Your neurosurgeon will discuss with you in advance which type of surgery you will have. On extremely rare occasions, this plan may need to change; however, if it does, your surgery will be rescheduled for another day.

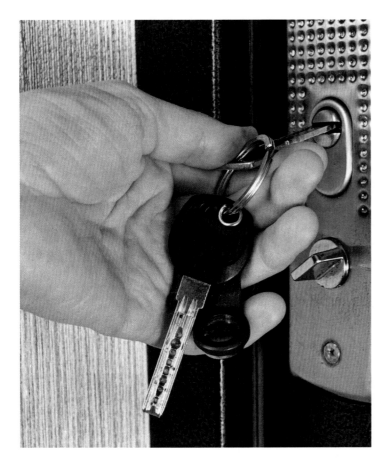

FRAME-BASED DBS

Originally, DBS surgery was done using a metal frame attached to the patient's head with four screws. Two of the screws go in the forehead and two in the back of the head. This ensures that the frame is fixed solidly to your head and will not move. The frame may be put on while you are asleep or while you are awake. The surgeon will give you injections of a medicine, usually lidocaine, in your scalp to make the areas where the screws will go in numb. The purposes of this frame are to help the surgeon find the spot to put the DBS electrode into your brain and to hold your head very still during surgery.

With this procedure, you will come to the hospital very early in the morning on the day of your surgery and have the frame attached to your head by your surgeon or someone on the surgical team. Then, you will have a CT scan and/or an MRI while wearing the frame. Often, you will travel on a rolling stretcher to the radiology department for this scan; however, some centers have a portable CT scanner in the operating room (O-arm® or CereTom®), so a scan can be done without moving you to another place.

Then, the surgeon will spend a few minutes creating the "plan" for your surgery. What this means is that the surgeon will look at your MRI and CT scans and then will determine the best spot to place the DBS electrode in your brain and where to make the cut on your head and the opening in your skull. Then the surgeon will attach your head frame to the operating-room table and make adjustments to it based on the information he or she got during planning. Frame-based DBS surgery is still widely used today in the US and internationally. If a frame is used, it will be removed after your surgery is done, before you wake up.

In the last several years, two companies have developed what are known as "frameless" DBS systems. They were designed for two purposes: first, to make the procedure more comfortable for patients, and second, to shorten the procedure time by eliminating the need to get another MRI or CT scan on the day of surgery. The two systems are slightly different but have major similarities. With both systems, you will have tiny screws put in your skull. One system, FHC's STarFix™, requires you to have the screws put in your skull a week before your surgery. This may be done in the doctor's office or in the operating room and may be done with you awake or asleep, depending on the what the surgeon prefers. It is usually a procedure with very little pain.

If you are awake, the surgeon will give you injections of medicine, such as lidocaine, to numb the area in which the screws will be placed. Then, the surgeon will make a tiny incision in your scalp with a knife and use a power screwdriver to fix the screws into your skull. The screws only go through the outer layers of your skull and do not get anywhere near your brain. The surgeon will then put a stitch or staple in the skin over the screw, so the screw will be completely underneath your skin. Then you will have a CT scan, and the surgeon will make the "plan" for your surgery at that time. The surgeon then sends the plan to a company to create a small "platform" that is custom-made for your head. The platform is made on a 3D printer. The tiny screws, which are about 2 mm in size, will stay in your head until the day of your brain surgery. Most people have minor pain from this that gets better with acetaminophen (Tylenol).

On the day of surgery, once you are in the operating room the platform will be attached to the screws in your head. This platform serves the same purpose as the metal frame—it is built to give the surgeon the exact spots to make the cut in your head and place the electrode in your brain. The other system, Medtronic's NexFrame®, does not require the screws to be put in your skull until the day of surgery. This system uses an adjustable "miniframe" that attaches to the skull screws. With both frameless systems, the screws are removed after the electrodes are placed in your brain and before you wake up from surgery.

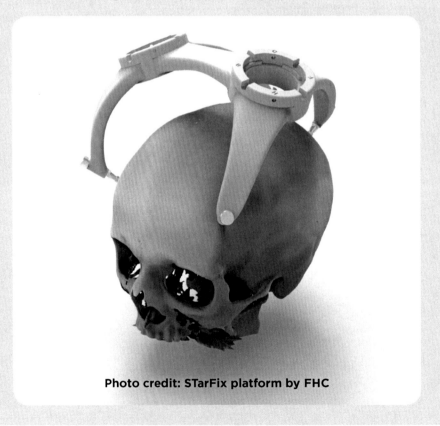

Photo credit: STarFix platform by FHC

AWAKE DBS

Why do I need to be awake during surgery?

Whether you have a frame-based or frameless system, your neurosurgeon may choose to keep you awake during part of your DBS surgery. There are two reasons for this. The first reason is to make sure that the DBS will control your tremor. While you are awake, the surgeon will "test" the electrode in your brain by sending a small bit of electricity through it. When this electricity reaches the right spot in your brain, your tremor will stop. The second reason is to check to see if you are having side effects from DBS. Some of the side effects, like tingling and changes to your speech, can only be checked while you are awake.

Who is in the operating room?

Depending on the type of hospital at which you have your surgery, there may be between five and 20 people in the operating room. This can seem overwhelming if you are not ready for it. Ask your surgeon during your pre-operative visit (the last office visit before your surgery) to tell you who will be in the operating room with you during your surgery. Typically, this includes your surgeon and at least one assistant to the surgeon. The assistant could be a resident, who is a doctor in training; a physician's assistant (PA), who has four years of schooling similar to medical school; or a surgical technician, who could be a nurse or skilled worker trained to help with surgery.

There will also be an anesthesiologist, who will give you medicine to relax you during the surgery and who will make sure that you are breathing well and that your blood pressure stays normal during the surgery. This person will also give you pain medicine if you are having pain when you wake up during the surgery. The anesthesiologist usually has at least one helper, and the two of them will usually take turns taking care of you during the surgery. So the person there when you go to sleep in the beginning of your surgery may not be the same person you see when you wake up.

WHAT IS IT LIKE TO BE AWAKE DURING SURGERY?

It may sound scary to be awake for even part of your surgery. But most people actually stay very calm for a few reasons. First, the brain itself does not feel pain! You may feel some discomfort from the screws of the frame or platform, and you may experience some back or neck pain from the position you will be in while lying on the operating-room table. Often, small adjustments can be made to help ease this pain, or the anesthesiologist may be able to give you a little pain medicine at a certain point during the surgery. Second, your doctors will be talking to you the entire time that you are awake. They will be asking you questions and talking you through what is going on. Third, in most cases you will only be awake for about 30 minutes to an hour.

There will be a nurse or assistant who will be handing the operating tools, like the knife, drill, and stitches, to the surgeon. This person may also change during the procedure. There will also be a nurse who is "circulating" in the room. This person's role is to make sure the surgeon and anesthesiologist have everything they need for the surgery. He or she may come in and out of the operating room several times during your surgery. This person may also change in the middle of your surgery, when another nurse comes in to give the first nurse a break. A neurologist may or may not be in the operating room with you, depending on the center at which you have the surgery. This may be your neurologist, or someone you have not met before; not all neurologists are trained to help neurosurgeons during DBS surgery.

There will also be a technician to run the equipment that "tests" the electrodes to make sure they are in the right spot. At some points during the surgery, a radiology technician may bring in x-ray equipment to help the surgeon check the location of the electrodes after they are placed in your brain. Usually there is also someone from the DBS company that makes the electrodes that will be put in your brain. If you are having a "frameless" procedure, someone from the company that makes your DBS platform may be there, too. Finally, there sometimes may be a medical student or other observers who are there to learn about the surgery you are having. This will usually be limited to one or two people, depending on the decision of the neurosurgeon.

What happens in the operating room?

Typically, when you are brought into the operating room, the anesthesiologist gives you medicine through an intravenous line or "IV," which is a tube that is inserted through a needle into a vein in your arm, hand, or foot. This medicine will make you very sleepy. You will also have either a mask placed over your nose and mouth or a small tube placed in your nose to give you oxygen so you can breathe. Once you are asleep, you may have other IVs put in and possibly a catheter in your bladder (to collect urine). Then, the surgeon will start the surgery. While you are asleep, the surgeon will make a cut or cuts in your head, attach the platform to the screws in your head (if you have a frameless procedure), drill a hole or holes in your skull, and open the lining that protects the brain.

The cuts in your head will be located on the top of your head, usually close to your hairline, and may be cut in a straight line or curved. The holes that are drilled are about the size of a nickel but may be smaller, depending on the surgeon's preference. Keep in mind that the DBS electrode is placed on the *opposite* side of your brain from the arm or leg that has the tremor. This is because the brain pathways crisscross at the bottom of the skull before they go into the spinal cord. So if you have a tremor in your left arm, the DBS electrode will be placed on the right side of your brain. The surgeon will then place one or more (up to five) very small metal tubes into your brain slowly and then put in the electrodes through the tube or tubes.

At this point, the anesthesiologist will usually wake you up from surgery. Many neurosurgeons choose to use microelectrode recording (MER) to help them find the best spot in your brain to place the DBS electrode. In this case, the electrodes they first put into your brain are very tiny. These electrodes are used to record the sounds your brain cells make. By listening to the pattern of sounds your brain cells make, the neurosurgeon and/or neurologist is able to tell where each electrode is in your brain. Next, the neurologist or surgeon will start gently moving around your arms and legs and will lightly touch your arms, legs, face, and tongue with a cotton swab while listening to your brain cells. If an electrode is in the right location to control your tremor, your brain cells will make a different sound when your body is moved or lightly touched.

Once the surgeon finds the perfect spot, he or she will take the microelectrode(s) out and put the DBS electrode into your head through the metal tube. Then, they will "test" the electrode by sending electricity through it. You may feel some tingling in your arms, legs, or face during this time. This is normal. You may also feel a tightening or pulling sensation in your arms, legs, or face, or have trouble speaking. This is a side effect of stimulation. If this feeling is intense, your surgeon may choose to move the electrode to a slightly different spot and then test it again. Sometimes, surgeons want to turn up the electricity high enough until they actually find side effects. This will help them when they program the DBS system later to set it at safe levels.

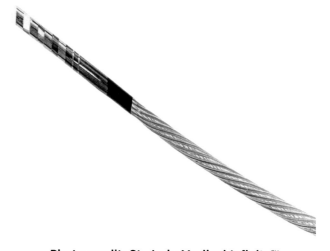

**Photo credit: St. Jude Medical Infinity™
segmented 1.5 directional lead by Abbott**

At this point, the doctor will also check to see how well your tremor is controlled. You may be asked to do some of the same things you did during your evaluation with the doctor before surgery. This includes touching your finger to your doctor's finger and then to your chin. It may include holding an empty cup out in front of you and bringing it back and forth towards your mouth. It may involve writing your name on a paper and drawing a spiral. You will be asked to do these things twice during the surgery. The first time you will do it is before the electrode is placed. Expect to see your normal amount of tremor at this point. Then, you will be asked to do these things again once the electrode is in your brain and electricity is running through it. This is often a very emotional moment for people. You finally get a glimpse of what life can be like without tremor.

The goal of electrode testing is not to make the system "perfect"; you may still have some tremor. The goal is to have the electrode placed in an area that is "safe," meaning it is unlikely to cause severe side effects, and to have it be "programmable," meaning that the DBS system can be adjusted later to control your tremor by at least 90%. Once the surgeon is happy with where the electrode is, he or she will then lock it in place, using a little plastic cap that is screwed into your skull with tiny screws. The electrode should not be able to move once the cap is on. If you are having two electrodes placed, the same procedure will be repeated on the other side of your head. Usually, the surgeon will have drilled both holes in your head before they wake you up to test the electrode, so this keeps the time you are awake to 30 minutes to an hour for one electrode and 1 to 1½ hours for two electrodes. The total surgery time is usually between 2½ and 5 hours.

After the electrodes are placed, you will be put to sleep for the rest of the surgery, and the surgeon will put stitches or staples in your head. Keep in mind that the end of the electrode is buried underneath the skin

and not attached to anything at the moment, so do not expect to see any changes in your tremor at this point. However, some people do have a temporary effect from placing the electrodes, and tremors can be reduced anywhere from mildly to completely. This effect usually wears off after a few hours or days and is therefore called the "honeymoon effect." When you wake up from surgery, you may or may not remember being awake during surgery. This is different for each patient.

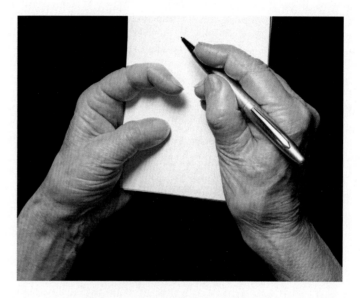

I remember the first DBS surgery I saw when I was a resident. The patient was about 72 years old and had a tremor that was so bad, she couldn't read her writing. All she wanted from the surgery was to be able to write letters to her friends so they could read them. During the surgery, I watched as she scribbled her name on the paper, and it was true—it was impossible to read. Then, the surgeon turned on the electricity to the DBS, and she was asked to write again. What I saw was something amazing. When she put her pen to paper, she wrote her name beautifully, legibly, and she began to cry tears of joy. That was a miracle in my eyes. That was a defining moment in my life. That is the reason I became a neurosurgeon who specializes in treating patients like you, who have tremor.

Who can have DBS surgery without being awake?

A DBS surgery may be done while you are asleep for a number of reasons:

- *Surgeon preference*
- *Patient's medical condition makes it unsafe to have surgery awake (e.g., severe breathing problems, extreme nervousness, dystonia/jerking movements when awake)*
- *To make it easier on the patient to have both parts of the surgery on the same day*

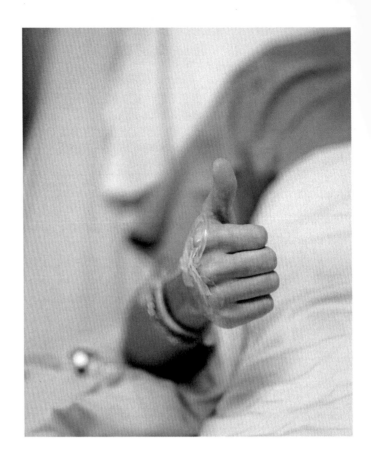

Generally, it will not be up to you whether you have surgery asleep or awake, although some centers may offer this choice in certain cases.

HOW CAN THE SURGEON MAKE SURE THE ELECTRODES ARE IN THE RIGHT PLACE IF I'M ASLEEP?

Most surgeons who do DBS surgery while you are asleep will use an MRI machine during the surgery. In this way, they are able to "see" where the electrodes are in the brain by looking at an image of your brain taken with the MRI. There are two main ways surgeons use MRIs to place your electrodes. In certain hospitals, there are MRI "suites" that are actually operating rooms in which an MRI can be slid in and out of the room on ceiling rollers. These are called "IMRIS" (intraoperative MRI suite) surgeries. You usually will be put to sleep before you ever go into these rooms and will wake up when you are back in the recovery room.

The surgery is done in a similar way to awake DBS surgery (described above), except that the recording electrodes are generally not used. Once the electrodes are in your brain, you will have an MRI, and your surgeon can look at them to see if they are in the right spot. Occasionally, your surgeon will also be able to test for side effects from stimulation without waking you up. Your surgeon will not be able to tell if you have side effects like tingling but will know if you have a muscle that tightens during testing. In this case, the electrode would be moved. In hospitals that do not have an IMRIS, you may still be able to have DBS in one of the rooms in the radiology department with an MRI, in which surgeries can be done in the same room. There are special safety rules that have to be followed in order to do this, so not all hospitals offer this as an option.

The second way an MRI can be used to place your DBS electrodes is by using the Clear-Point® system. This involves a disposable plastic frame that is attached to your head after you go to sleep. Then a computerized system is used to adjust the frame so that your electrodes can be placed in the exact spot determined by your surgeon.

What happens after surgery?

For any of the above procedures, you will wake up from surgery in the operating room and then go to the recovery room for an hour or two before being admitted to the hospital. The reason you go to the recovery room first is that if there is a major problem, such as you have trouble breathing or start bleeding from the surgery, this will often happen in the first couple of hours after surgery. In the recovery room, you have a nurse watching you closely to make sure no problems occur. Sometimes, a doctor will order a CT scan and/or x-rays while you are in the recovery room to make sure the electrodes are in a good position in your brain and that you are not having bleeding into the brain. You will move to a hospital room once the doctors and nurses say it is safe for you to leave the recovery room, and you will spend at least one night, possibly two or more, in the hospital. Most people go home the morning after surgery. There is not much pain with this surgery. You should be able to take acetaminophen (Tylenol) to control the pain. Once you go home from the hospital, you should take it easy for about a week. You generally will not need someone to stay at home with you, and you should be able to take care of your basic needs, like eating and dressing, without help (provided you could do this before the surgery).

The second surgery

Most surgeons wait a few days to a couple of weeks before doing the second surgery to connect the DBS electrode(s) to the brain "pacemaker" that will be put in your chest. Some surgeons will do this part of the surgery right after the first part, especially if you had "asleep surgery" for the first part. This second surgery is much shorter than the first, lasting less than an hour. You will be asleep for the whole procedure, and you will go home after you spend an hour or two in the recovery room. Your surgeon will make a small cut on your head where the end of the electrode is and then another cut just below your collarbone, about three inches in length. Your surgeon will run a connecting wire from the brain electrode(s) to the

pacemaker. This is done using a tool that makes a "tunnel" just under the skin of your neck.

Once everything is attached, your surgeon will put in stitches or staples, and you will wake up and go to the recovery room. Everything is placed under the skin, just like with the first part of the surgery, so no wires or other parts of the system will be visible. You may be able to feel the wire in your neck, particularly if you are very thin. You will probably see a bulge and feel the pacemaker in your chest, although in time you will get used to it. If you shoot rifles regularly, or if you are an avid golfer, let your surgeon know before your surgery. You may need to have your pacemaker put in lower, in your belly area, so that it won't get in the way of your hobby, and so it will be protected.

Keep in mind that even though everything is hooked up, most of the time you will be home for a few weeks before the DBS system is turned on. This is because you could have a small amount of swelling in your brain after your electrodes are placed, and it can take a few weeks for the swelling to go down. Running electricity through a swollen brain can cause some side effects and can make it hard to find the right settings on the DBS system to control your tremor. You will come back to see your doctor to have the stitches from both surgeries taken out, usually about two weeks after the second surgery.

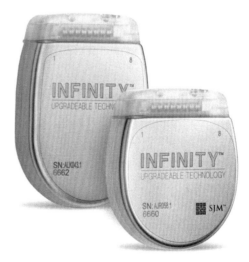

**Photo credit: St. Jude Medical Infinity™
IPG, 5 IPG, 7 IPG by Abbott**

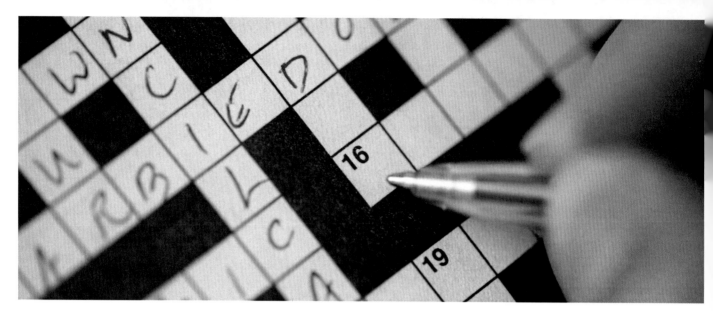

Programming and follow up

A few weeks after your DBS surgery, you will come into the office to have your first "programming" session done. This is usually the first time the DBS system will be turned on. Just like when the system is tested in the operating room, this can be an emotional moment for many people. When you have had a tremor for so long, seeing your hand steadier for the first time in years is often a very moving experience. The way the programming is done depends a lot on who is doing the programming and what kind of DBS system you have. Programming can be done by your surgeon, your movement disorder neurologist, another neurologist, or a physician's assistant. Anyone who is doing your programming should have gotten training to do this. Programming can take between a few minutes and a few hours.

Some doctors will test every contact on the electrode at different voltages (strengths of the electric current) to see what works best and what causes side effects. Others will use standard settings for the first programming session and only make changes if it does not work well or you have side effects that bother you a lot. The most common side effect is tingling in your arm, leg, or face. Other side effects include a pulling sensation in your arm, leg, or face, difficulty talking, or slurring your words. If you have those side effects, then your programming will be adjusted until you do

not experience them anymore. If your only side effect is tingling, but your tremor is well controlled, the programmer may leave the setting as it is. Tingling side effects usually get better in time, although in up to 20% of cases they do not get better.[4] In those cases, I have yet to see a patient who would rather have their tremor back just so the tingling would go away.

You should not expect your tremor to "stop" during this first programming session. Often it will decrease by about 50%, although a few people see a 90% decrease in tremor with the first programming. It may take you several months of programming sessions, coming in every few weeks, to find the best settings for your DBS. If, after a year, you are still not satisfied with the outcomes, you should talk to your surgeon about options for moving the electrode. Once you and your doctor are happy with your tremor control, you will only need to come in for appointments every six months or so. Your DBS leads should last indefinitely. You will have a CT or MRI scan between six months and one year after your DBS is placed, and will only need another scan if there is a problem with your system in the future. Your "pacemaker" will need to be replaced every two to three years if it has a standard battery or every five to seven years if it has a rechargeable battery. This is a very simple surgery that takes about 20 minutes, and you will be able to go home the same day after the surgery.

DBS systems decrease hand and arm tremors by as much as 80–90% in about 90% of people.[5-7] Those are some impressive results! You will see the most benefit in your hand and arm tremors, but occasionally your leg tremor will get better, too. If you have a voice or head tremor, you will need a DBS system on both sides of your head in order to have any improvement, and usually you only will see about a 50% decrease in these tremors. Importantly, the improvement you will see in your tremors after DBS does not depend on the type of the surgery you have. Both frame-based and frameless DBS systems are highly accurate—within 1–2 millimeters—as are awake and asleep methods of placing a DBS.[8-11] The DBS system will control your tremor for a long time—most people still have excellent tremor control after 10 years.[5]

The most common complication in DBS surgeries is infection. You have about a 2–5% risk of getting an infection with DBS.[5,12] A much rarer but more serious complication is bleeding in the brain, or having a stroke. This happens in fewer than 1 out of 100 people. When it happens, sometimes it is very small, and you would not even know it happened unless your doctor had a CT scan of your brain. In some cases, a stroke can cause temporary or permanent problems, like weakness on one side of your body or difficulty speaking or understanding words. In extreme cases, you may need another surgery to stop the bleeding or take out the blood clot to save your life.

Another complication that is uncommon and not as severe is that your electrodes or connecting wires may break. This happens more commonly the longer your electrodes have been in place (around 15-20 years). When the connecting wire between your electrode and pacemaker is broken, this is easily fixed with an outpatient surgery that lasts less than 30 minutes. When the brain wires break, this requires a new DBS electrode placement surgery. Finally, a rare side effect after DBS surgery is that you could have trouble speaking. This is most common if you are over the age of 70 and have two DBS leads placed during the same surgery.[13] For this reason, most neurosurgeons will place only one DBS lead at the time if you are over age 70, starting with the side with the worst tremor or with your dominant hand. Then, after a few months, if there are no surgical complications, you can have a second surgery to put in the other DBS lead.

Patients sometimes ask me if they can ever get an MRI again of their heads or other parts of their bodies after they have DBS surgery. The answer is: It depends on the type of DBS system you have. Medtronic® systems that were placed around 2010 or later are generally MRI "compatible." This means that the MRI can safely be done in a place that has followed safety precautions for patients with DBS. Keep in mind that only certain hospitals and centers do this, so you cannot get your MRI anywhere you want. The other DBS systems (from Boston Scientific and St. Jude Medical/Abbott) do not have MRI-compatible electrodes at the time of this publication. Both companies expect to have MRI-compatible systems in the future.

Cost and insurance coverage

The cost of DBS varies greatly. In the US it can cost up to $65,000, depending on what type of DBS system you have and where you have the surgery.[14] Most insurance companies will cover DBS for tremors, if your tremor is bad enough. Your doctor usually will need to prove to your insurance company that your tremor interferes with your daily activities, such as eating, dressing, and writing, or affects your ability to work. In general, insurance companies want to see that your tremor has been classified as moderately severe to severe before they will pay for your surgery. You may have a co-pay or deductible (or both) that you will be responsible for paying.

What it is

Despite its name, the Gamma Knife procedure does not involve the use of a knife. Another name for this procedure is "stereotactic radiosurgery." Essentially, a Gamma Knife is a machine that creates a very tiny (4 mm) hole in your brain tissue using around 200 very low-intensity radiation beams. These beams all come from the machine at different angles and focus on the same point in your head. Creating this hole helps stop the "tremor cells" in your brain, which decreases your shaking. Each radiation beam has less radiation than you would get from standing out in the sun for a few minutes, so most of your brain will get very little radiation exposure. So you will not get the side effects you may have heard about people getting from "whole brain radiation" for cancer treatments.

WHO IS A CANDIDATE?

Almost anyone who has tremors should be able to have Gamma Knife treatment. The only reason you may not be able to have it is if you cannot get an MRI of your head for any reason (e.g., due to certain types of metal in your body from surgeries, an older pacemaker, etc.). As with DBS, you would only want to have this procedure if medicines and the other methods described in this book are not working well enough to control your tremor. Because Gamma Knife treatment often does not work as well as DBS to decrease tremors and because it will make a permanent hole in your brain, I often recommend Gamma Knife only if you cannot have DBS. For example, if you are not medically healthy enough for DBS surgery or have had too many infections after getting DBS, I would recommend Gamma Knife as an alternative.

What to expect

The entire Gamma Knife procedure usually takes about two hours. However, if you are having treatment at a center that does a lot of Gamma Knife procedures, you may spend the majority of a day at the center. When you come in for treatment, you may either go directly to get an MRI scan or see your doctor to have a "frame" placed on your head. This is the same type of frame described in the Deep Brain Stimulation section. Your doctor needs this frame on your head so that it will not move during the procedure. You do not want a hole in the wrong spot in your brain!

Your doctor will first give you some medicine to relax you. Then, your doctor will work with an assistant to place the metal frame on your head and will then give you four shots of medicine in your head—two in the forehead and two in the back of the head. Next, your doctor will put four screws in your head to hold the frame tightly. You will feel a lot of pressure while the screws are being put in, but if you feel pain, tell your doctor! They will give you more medicine to relax you, or they will give you more medicine to make those areas of your head numb. After this, you will have a CT scan of your head. If you did not have an MRI scan before the frame was placed, you will also have an MRI. After these scans, you will come back to the Gamma Knife center and wait for a period of time. During this time, your neurosurgeon will work with a radiation oncologist and a physicist to plan the perfect spot for the hole in your brain and to decide the right amount of radiation to safely make the hole without damaging other areas of your brain. The place where the hole will be in your brain may be different depending on whether your tremors are from ET or Parkinson's disease.

Once your treatment plan is made, which can take 30 minutes to an hour, you will be brought into the room with the Gamma Knife and laid down on a narrow table. The metal frame on your head will be attached to the table, and then the table will slide into the Gamma Knife machine. While you will be in the room by yourself, there will be cameras and a microphone in the room. There will be someone watching you and talking to you the entire time to make sure you are okay. If you start to feel anxious, speak up, and someone will come into the room to help you. You will be in the Gamma Knife for about an hour to an hour and a half.

When the procedure is finished, you will be taken off the table, and the metal frame will be taken off your head. You usually will be able to go home after another hour. Sometimes, your doctor will give you a medicine called a steroid that you will take for a few days. This can help with swelling in your brain. You should not feel much pain afterward. If you do have a headache in the day or two after the procedure, you can take acetaminophen (Tylenol) or ibuprofen (Advil, Motrin, etc.). If your pain lasts longer than two days, call your doctor.

Your first follow-up after Gamma Knife treatment may not be for another six months. At that time, you may have an MRI scan of your brain. This scan serves two purposes. First, it will show your surgeon that the hole in your brain is there and that it is the right size and in the right spot. Secondly, it will show your surgeon whether there is swelling in that area of your brain. You may have one more MRI a year after your Gamma Knife procedure if your surgeon thinks it is needed.

OUTCOMES AND COMPLICATIONS

Gamma Knife procedures typically decrease tremor caused by ET and Parkinson's disease in over 90% of patients.[15] Your arm and hand tremors should get at least 50% better and may get up to almost 90% better.[16,17] You may not get any relief from tremors in your leg, voice, or face. Gamma Knife treatment can also improve tremors caused by multiple sclerosis,[18] although this has not been studied as much. Keep in mind that it will take at least a month and possibly up to several months after your treatment before you see your tremor get better. This is because the Gamma Knife works using radiation, which takes time to create the hole in your brain. Over time, your tremor may also come back somewhat.[19]

There are very few complications from Gamma Knife surgery these days, as the treatment has been improved over time. One of the more common side effects you may have is a tingling feeling in the arm or leg that has been treated for tremor. Occasionally this feeling can be painful, although this is very rare. Even more rare is having weakness in your arm, leg, or face. If you have this procedure for tremors in both arms, a rare side effect is that you could have trouble talking clearly after surgery. This happens less than 5% of the time. Sometimes you may have side effects about six months after your procedure. If this happens, it is probably caused by swelling in your brain. The good news is, this will probably get better once you take a medicine known as a steroid for a few days. The reason it takes a few months to see side effects, if you have them, is that they are caused by the radiation, which takes about six months to fully set in.

Cost and insurance coverage

Gamma Knife treatment is less expensive than DBS surgery for a few reasons. First, you do not have to spend the night in the hospital, and you usually only need one treatment. You do not have to put permanent equipment in your head, which also lowers the cost. Most insurance companies will cover Gamma Knife treatment for your tremor. As with DBS, your insurance will approve this treatment if your tremor is bad enough to cause problems in your day-to-day life and if you have already tried taking many different medicines for your tremor.

What it is

Magnetic resonance-guided focused ultrasound (MRgFUS), also known as "Neuravive," is a newer procedure somewhat similar to Gamma Knife that creates a tiny hole in the brain that will help stop your shaking. It is different from Gamma Knife because it uses heat from an ultrasound (a machine using sound waves) instead of from radiation. An MRI is used to decide exactly where to place the hole. The other major difference between this and Gamma Knife surgery is that the ultrasound treatment will stop your tremor the same day, while Gamma Knife treatment can take a few months to work. Also, Gamma Knife surgery can be done on both sides of the head, while MRgFUS is currently only FDA approved to use on one side. If you have tremor on both sides of your body, your doctor will likely use MRgFUS to treat the arm with the worse tremor or the side that you use most often.

What to expect

The procedure takes anywhere from 2-3 hours. Before your MRgFUS procedure, you will usually have a CT scan of your head on the day of your treatment or a few days before. On the day of your treatment, you will have a metal frame attached to your head (just like for Gamma Knife and frame-based DBS). Then, you will lie down on a table in the MRI room. Your surgeon will talk to you throughout the procedure. First, a very low intensity of the ultrasound will be used to make a "test lesion." This is a temporary hole. Your doctor will then check to see if your tremor is getting better and if you are having any side effects. If your tremor has stopped and you are not having side effects, your surgeon will increase the intensity of the ultrasound and make the hole permanent. If you are having side effects or the tremor is not getting better, your doctor will do another test lesion in a different spot in your brain and check your tremor and side effects again. Your doctor will repeat this until he or she finds the perfect spot. Making these holes does not hurt.

WHO IS A CANDIDATE?

Because MRgFUS is not a "surgery," almost anyone who has tremors should be able to have this treatment. The only reason you may not be able to have this procedure is if you cannot get an MRI of your head. As with all of the treatments described in this chapter, you should only have this procedure if medicines and other methods do not sufficiently control your tremor. Because ultrasound often does not work as well as DBS to decrease tremors and because it makes a permanent hole in your brain, I typically recommend MRgFUS only if you cannot get DBS due to medical or psychological reasons.

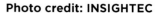

Photo credit: INSIGHTEC

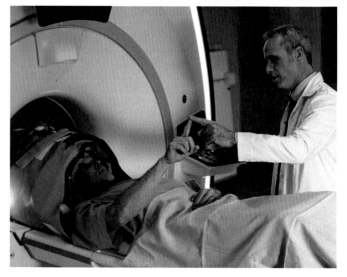

Once the procedure is finished, you will be taken off the MRI table and the frame will be taken off of your head. You will not have to wait for the treatment to work—your tremor will be controlled at this point. After a short period of time, you will be able to go home. You should not have much of a headache after this procedure. If you do, it should last only a day or two. Please call your doctor if your pain lasts longer than this. You will likely have a couple of follow-up visits with your doctor in several months as well as an MRI scan.

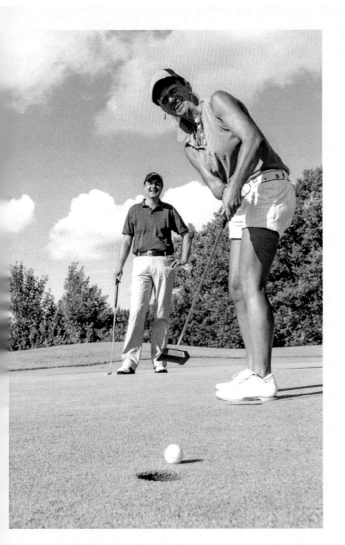

MRgFUS treatment decreases tremor in about 35%-80% of patients.[2,20,21] As described above, your tremor will get better as soon as your treatment is finished.[22] As with Gamma Knife surgery, some tremor will come back in about a third of people who have MRgFUS treatment.[20] It is possible to have side effects from this treatment; however, severe side effects such as weakness are not very likely, since your doctor will have done a test lesion to check for side effects. The most common side effects are a tingling feeling in your arms or legs, which could be painful, and mild difficulty walking.[2]

Cost and insurance coverage

The cost of MRgFUS is similar to the cost of Gamma Knife and significantly lower than the cost of DBS.[23] Because MRgFUS is a relatively new procedure, some insurance companies may not cover it. Medicare, however, usually will cover MRgFUS treatment for tremors due to ET or Parkinson's disease.

RADIOFREQUENCY ABLATION

What it is

Radiofrequency (RF) ablation or lesioning, also called "stereotactic thalamotomy," is similar in some ways to Gamma Knife and MRgFUS treatment. It creates a small hole in the brain to slow down or stop tremors, and, like ultrasound treatment, improves your tremor right after the procedure is done. The major difference between RF ablation and these other treatments is that RF ablation requires brain surgery. It can also control tremor much better than Gamma Knife and ultrasound treatments.

WHO IS A CANDIDATE?

RF ablation was the go-to surgery for people with tremors before DBS was approved to treat tremors in 1997. Most neurosurgeons now will recommend DBS before considering RF ablation. Both procedures require you to be a good candidate for surgery, but we prefer to use a therapy that is reversible and adjustable, like DBS. RF ablation, on the other hand, is irreversible. Your doctor may recommend RF ablation to you if you are healthy enough for surgery but have any of the following issues: you do not want objects implanted in your brain; you do not want to come back to the office for programming appointments; or you have had infections with DBS and need to have the DBS system removed. In the last case, your surgeon can do the RF ablation in the same surgery as DBS removal.

The procedure for RF ablation is similar in many ways to DBS surgery. Most surgeons who do RF ablation use a frame-based system (see above). You will have a metal frame attached to your head and will have a CT scan after the frame is placed. Then you will be brought into the operating room and given medicine to relax you. The next parts of the surgery are the same as DBS surgery, up to and including the microelectrode recording. After this, your surgeon will place a probe in your brain and send an electric current through the end of the probe until it makes a small hole in your brain. Your surgeon will test your tremor to see how much better it has gotten and will also check for side effects. If your tremor is well controlled at this point, your surgeon will take out the probe and put stitches in your head. If you still have a lot of tremors, your surgeon may put a hole in another nearby spot in your brain.

After surgery, you will go to a recovery room, where you will be watched for an hour or two. Then you will be admitted to the hospital overnight. You should be able to go home the next morning. Your tremor will be better as soon as the surgery is done, and you should not have very much pain. You should take it easy for about a week after the surgery. Your surgeon will probably want to see you a couple weeks after surgery to take out your stitches. Then, you will only need to see your surgeon a couple more times to check your wounds and possibly have an MRI or CT scan.

OUTCOMES AND COMPLICATIONS

RF ablation generally works very well to control your tremors. Studies show that this procedure will almost completely get rid of your tremors.[24] Side effects from RF ablation are the same as from DBS, including infection, bleeding in the brain, weakness, and tingling or numbness in your arms, legs, or face. If you are going to have side effects, they will happen within the first 24-48 hours after your surgery.

Cost and insurance coverage

The cost of RF ablation is less than DBS surgery but more than Gamma Knife or MRgFUS treatment. RF ablation requires an overnight hospital stay and use of an operating room, which increases the cost. However, unlike DBS, you will have nothing implanted in your brain. Most insurance companies will cover the cost of RF ablation to treat tremor due to ET or Parkinson's disease.

Outcomes comparison

Procedure	Tremor decrease	Surgery?	When tremor stops	Tremor control over time	Reversible
DBS	50-90%	Yes	1 mo. after surgery	Very good	Yes
Gamma Knife	40-80%	No	6 mo.–1 yr.	Good	No
MRgFUS	40-90%	No	Immediately	Not known[25]	No
RF ablation	80-100%	Yes	Immediately	Good	No

REFERENCES

1. Benabid AL, Pollak P, Louveau A, Henry S, de Rougemont J. Combined (thalamotomy and stimulation) stereotactic surgery of the VIM thalamic nucleus for bilateral Parkinson disease. *Appl Neurophysiol.* 1987;50(1-6):344–346.

2. Mohammed N, Patra D, Nanda A. A meta-analysis of outcomes and complications of magnetic resonance-guided focused ultrasound in the treatment of essential tremor. *Neurosurg Focus.* 2018;44(2):E4.

3. Ishikita T, Ishiguro A, Fujisawa K, Tsukimoto I, Shimbo T. Carbamazepine-induced thrombocytopenia defined by a challenge test. *Am J Hematol.* 1999;62(1):52-5.

4. Deuschl G, Herzog J, Kleiner-Fisman G, et al. Deep brain stimulation: postoperative issues. *Mov Disord.* 2006;21(suppl 14):S219-37.

5. Cury RG, Fraix V, Castrioto A, et al. Thalamic deep brain stimulation for tremor in Parkinson disease, essential tremor, and dystonia. *Neurology.* 2017;89(13):1416-1423.

6. Bryant JA, De Salles A, Cabatan C, Frysinger R, Behnke E, Bronstein J. The impact of thalamic stimulation on activities of daily living for essential tremor. *Surg Neurol.* 2003;59:479–485.

7. Pahwa R, Lyons KE, Wilkinson SB, et al. Long-term evaluation of deep brain stimulation of the thalamus. *J Neurosurg.* 2006;104(4):506-12.

8. Bot M, van den Munckhof P, Bakay R, Sierens D, Stebbins G, Verhagen Metman L. Analysis of stereotactic accuracy in patients undergoing deep brain stimulation using Nexframe and the Leksell Frame. *Stereotact Funct Neurosurg.* 2015;93(5):316-25.

9. Chabardes S, Isnard S, Castrioto A, et al. Surgical implantation of STN-DBS leads using intraoperative MRI guidance: technique, accuracy, and clinical benefit at 1-year follow-up. *Acta Neurochir (Wien).* 2015;157(4):729-37.

10. Konrad PE, Neimat JS, Yu H, et al. Customized, miniature rapid-prototype stereotactic frames for use in deep brain stimulator surgery: initial clinical methodology and experience from 263 patients from 2002 to 2008. *Stereotact Funct Neurosurg.* 2011;89(1):34-41.

11. Ostrem JL, Ziman N, Galifianakis NB, et al. Clinical outcomes using ClearPoint interventional MRI for deep brain stimulation lead placement in Parkinson's disease. *J Neurosurg.* 2016;124(4):908-16.

12. Verla T, Marky A, Farber H, et al. Impact of advancing age on post-operative complications of deep brain stimulation surgery for essential tremor. *J Clin Neurosci.* 2015;22(5):872-6.

13. Fields JA, Tröster AI, Woods SP, et al. Neuropsychological and quality of life outcomes 12 months after unilateral thalamic stimulation for essential tremor. J Neurol Neurosurg Psychiatry. 2003;74(3):305-11.

14. Rossi PJ, Giordano J, Okun MS. The problem of funding off-label deep brain stimulation. bait-and-switch tactics and the need for policy reform. *JAMA Neurol.* 2017;74(1):9-10.

15. Witjas T, Carron R, Boutin E, Eusebio A, Azulay JP, Régis J. Essential tremor: update of therapeutic strategies (medical treatment and gamma knife thalamotomy). *Rev Neurol (Paris).* 2016;172(8-9):408-415.

16. Raju SS, Niranjan A, Monaco Iii EA, Flickinger JC, Lunsford LD. Stereotactic radiosurgery for intractable tremor-dominant Parkinson disease: a retrospective analysis. *Stereotact Funct Neurosurg.* 2017;95(5):291-297.

17. Niranjan A, Raju SS, Kooshkabadi A, Monaco E 3rd, Flickinger JC, Lunsford LD. Stereotactic radiosurgery for essential tremor: retrospective analysis of a 19-year experience. *Mov Disord.* 2017;32(5):769-777.

18. Raju SS, Niranjan A, Monaco EA 3rd, Flickinger JC, Lunsford LD. Stereotactic radiosurgery for medically refractory multiple sclerosis-related tremor. *J Neurosurg.* Jun 2017:1-8.

19. Niranjan A, Jawahar A, Kondziolka D, Lunsford LD. A comparison of surgical approaches for the management of tremor: radiofrequency thalamotomy, gamma knife thalamotomy and thalamic stimulation. *Stereotact Funct Neurosurg.* 1999;72:178–184

20. Elias WJ, Huss D, Voss T, et al. A pilot study of focused ultrasound thalamotomy for essential tremor. *N Engl J Med.* 2013;369:640–648.

21. Chang WS, Jung HH, Zadicario E, et al. Factors associated with successful magnetic resonance-guided focused ultrasound treatment: efficiency of acoustic energy delivery through the skull. *J Neurosurg.* 2016;124:411–416.

22. Chang WS, Jung HH, Kweon EJ, Zadicario E, Rachmilevitch I, Chang JW. Unilateral magnetic resonance guided focused ultrasound thalamotomy for essential tremor: practices and clinicoradiological outcomes. *J Neurol Neurosurg Psychiatry.* 2015;86(3):257-64.

23. Ravikumar VK, Parker JJ, Hornbeck TS, et al. Cost-effectiveness of focused ultrasound, radiosurgery, and DBS for essential tremor. *Mov Disord.* 2017;32(8):1165-1173.

24. Kim M, Jung NY, Park CK, Chang WS, Jung HH, Chang JW. Comparative evaluation of magnetic resonance-guided focused ultrasound surgery for essential tremor. *Stereotact Funct Neurosurg.* 2017;95(4):279-286.

25. Rohani M, Fasano A. Focused ultrasound for essential tremor: review of the evidence and discussion of current hurdles. *Tremor Other Hyperkinet Mov (N Y).* 2017;7:462.

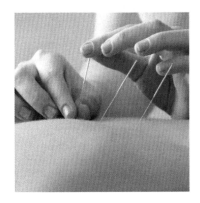
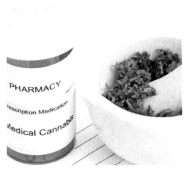
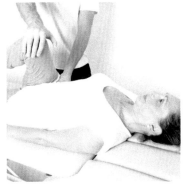
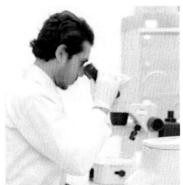
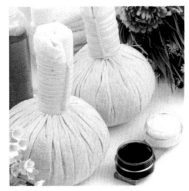
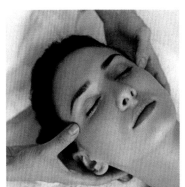
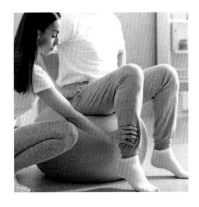
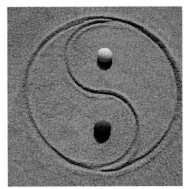
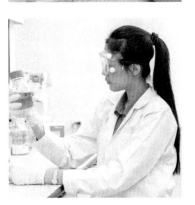

SECTION

4

ALTERNATIVE
TREATMENTS
AND RESEARCH

ALTERNATIVE TREATMENTS

You may not realize that there are a variety of alternative treatments that can help reduce your tremors. Most doctors do not know about these, so you may have never heard that they can be helpful. As with all treatments, consider talking to your doctor before starting any of these programs, and listen to your body! If something is causing you pain, or if you start having new symptoms, then take a break from the therapy and see if your symptoms get better.

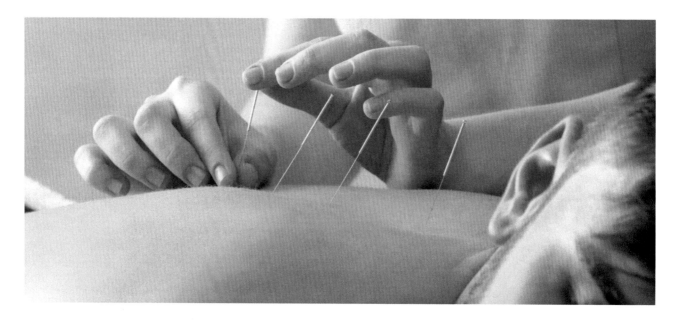

ACUPUNCTURE

What it is and how it works

The origin of acupuncture treatment is debated. It may have started as far back as 5000 years ago in ancient Egypt, as some hieroglyphics suggest that needles were being used. Others say that acupuncture started in China 2000 years ago. Acupuncture involves inserting tiny needles into specific places in the body in order to treat illness or relieve pain. The needles are extremely thin—about as thick as a strand of hair—and range from about a half-inch to five inches long. They are sterilized and, at least in the US, are never reused. The needles usually go only a few millimeters into the skin, although this depends on where on the body the needles are placed. Some needles put into fat tissue can go in as much as four inches.

It is difficult to explain exactly how acupuncture works in a few words. You will get different explanations depending on whether you ask a "traditional" or "modern" acupuncturist. The general idea behind acupuncture involves helping the "vital energy" in your body, also known as Qi (pronounced "chee"), to flow better so that your body gets back into balance or harmony. The idea of Qi can be difficult to understand; it is something that you can feel but not see. Think of how you feel when you are driving behind a smog-filled truck making a lot of noise. That feeling is similar to Qi that is out of balance. Now think of yourself walking along the beach or in the woods during a peaceful moment. That feeling is similar to Qi that is in balance. Acupuncture works by getting you closer to that second feeling. You can also think of acupuncture as a way to trigger nerves and chemicals in your body to help heal you.

Acupuncturists often work in centers or medical offices with other medical professionals. They occasionally work in chiropractic offices, as these services can work well when done together. Acupuncturists may also be in centers for "integrative" or "holistic" medicine or in "mind-body" centers or centers for "Eastern medicine." There are also a number of other centers in which you may find an acupuncturist. Importantly, you should look for an acupuncturist who is licensed by your state's medical board.

Once you find an acupuncturist, look up his or her name on your state's medical license website, which you can easily find with an internet search. You will be able to see whether your acupuncturist has an active license to practice acupuncture and sometimes also how long he or she has been in practice. You can also look up reviews posted by patients, although keep in mind that people are more likely to post negative than positive reviews—so take these with a grain of salt.

Lastly, when you have your first visit with your acupuncturist, you should ask about training—did he or she train in China or locally? What certification does he or she have? The highest acupuncture certification comes from the National Certification Commission. Their website (www.nccaom.org) has a section called "Find a Practitioner" that can also help you locate an acupuncturist. Your acupuncturist should have had a minimum of 1700 hours of training and should have a solid understanding of pulses and tongue examination. These are critical parts of your exam that help your acupuncturist figure out the best treatment for you. Also ask how many years your acupuncturist has been practicing and whether he or she can give you references. Importantly, ask your acupuncturist if he or she has experience treating tremors. Not all training programs focus on teaching these techniques.

DOES IT HURT?

The first question most people have about acupuncture is, "Does it hurt?" The answer is: not very much. Most people find acupuncture to be completely painless, even while the needles are going in. Some people experience a quick, mild "pricking" sensation just as a needle goes in. After all the needles are in, they should not hurt at all if they are well placed. It can still be a scary idea, though, that someone will be putting needles into your body! As someone who receives acupuncture treatments on a regular basis, I can still remember the first time I had a treatment. How could I, as a doctor, be scared of a medical treatment, you ask? Well, you are talking to someone who has no problem cutting into other people's heads but has to have a nurse hold my hand while my own blood is being drawn! I remember asking one of my friends to come with me to my first acupuncture appointment and to sit with me and hold my hand while the needles were going in. I was so scared, but the truth is, it was not bad at all. Now when I go, on some days my skin is more sensitive than on other days, so I have learned a few tricks to help me during these times.

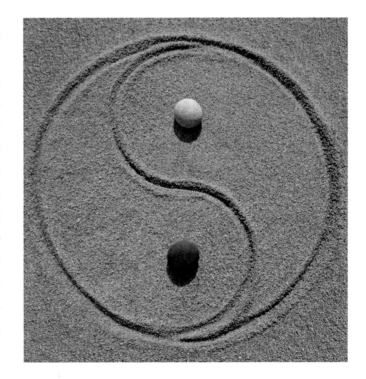

Tips and tricks

1. Take deep breaths: I practice deep breathing while the needles are being placed. I find if I take a deep breath in just before the needle goes in, and then breathe out slowly as it is being inserted, I feel no pain.

2. Meditate: Sometimes I listen to meditations on my phone while the needles are going in. Sometimes I think about something positive, like a vacation I have recently taken or one I am planning. Distraction is a great tool!

3. Listen to music: Your acupuncturist will likely have soothing music playing in the room. If not, you often can bring your own music to listen to with in-ear headphones. (These usually do not get in the way of the needles.)

4. Change order of placement: Have your acupuncturist put in certain needles first to help keep you calm. There are certain areas, particularly on the scalp, in the ears, or on the wrist, that give you an almost immediate sense of calm when a needle is placed there.

5. Speak up: If you have more than a couple of seconds of pain after any needle is put in, ask to have it adjusted slightly! Sometimes the needles can touch a nerve or blood vessel that can cause pain until the needle is moved.

6. Ask for a short break: If you are really nervous while the needles are going in, then ask your acupuncturist to give you a short break before putting in the next needle. Sometimes a couple of breaths in between needles can really help you be less nervous!

What to expect

Usually acupuncture appointments are scheduled for one hour. Of that time, you will likely spend 30-40 minutes with the needles inserted in your skin. First you will have a short (5-10 minute) consultation with your acupuncturist. This may be longer during your first visit. Your acupuncturist will ask all about your medical history. Tell your acupuncturist about all your health issues, not just what you are there to have treated. There are many spots needles can be placed to treat the same condition. Often your acupuncturist's choice of the best spots for your condition will change based on other medical problems or psychological problems (e.g., depression, nervousness) you have. Next, you will lie down on a cushioned table. The table may be heated. You can also ask to have the temperature adjusted to make you more comfortable.

You will be completely dressed for most visits with your acupuncturist, unless needles need to be placed in your back or stomach area. It is helpful if you can wear loose clothing, because your sleeves or pants legs may need to be rolled up to place needles in the lower parts of your legs, below your knees, or in your wrists or lower parts of your arms. Your acupuncturist will then check the pulses in both of your arms and will look at your tongue. This gives him or her information about how your body is functioning overall. Your acupuncturist will use this information to help diagnose you and figure out where you may need needles placed. He or she may ask you questions while doing this (such as if you have had a cold recently) to help make these decisions.

NEEDLE PLACEMENT AND TREATMENT

Next, your acupuncturist will clean areas of your skin where the needles will be placed with alcohol. You may have only a few needles placed, or it may be more than 20. You can ask your acupuncturist before he or she starts how many needles will be used, so you will know when they are all in. Once all the needles are in place, you may be covered with a light sheet or blanket. Some acupuncturists have a space heater that can be directed at your feet if your socks are off. Then, your acupuncturist will usually leave the room and turn off the lights. Try not to move much while the needles are in place. You can slightly move your hands or your feet or adjust your back a little to make yourself more comfortable.

If you have back pain, you may find that a small pillow under your knees or back helps you lie still for the treatment. You may fall asleep once the needles are in place. This is fine, and you will get the same benefit as you would if you were awake. I usually use the time to meditate. If you stay awake, you may have "tingling" feelings moving throughout your body. This is totally normal and nothing to worry about. Your acupuncturist will likely check on you after 10-15 minutes. At this time, he or she may twist the needles to make them go slightly deeper into your skin. This should not hurt. Then your acupuncturist will often leave the room again for another 15-20 minutes. When your acupuncturist comes back, he or she will gradually brighten the lights and then remove the needles.

REMOVAL AND FOLLOW UP

Removal should not hurt. Sometimes your acupuncturist may dab some ointment over the areas where the needles were removed. You often will be asked how you feel. You may have a sense of calmness or peace. You may also get a little light headed, so take your time sitting up. Then, you will be asked to schedule a follow-up appointment. Your treatments may be weekly or every other week for the first two to three months. After that, treatments can often be spread out to a few times per year. Acupuncturists may also use other methods, in addition to placing needles, to treat you. Some of these methods, such as cupping, have not been studied formally for the treatment of essential tremor (ET) and Parkinson's disease, but anecdotally they help reduce tremors in both conditions.

Cost and insurance coverage

Acupuncture treatments usually range in cost from about $40 to $80 per session. Sometimes packages are offered that lower your cost per visit if you buy three to five visits at once. Some insurances will cover the cost of acupuncture, although this is uncertain, particularly if you are going to receive the treatment for tremors. If you happen to have pain in your back or somewhere else in your body, you have a much better chance of having your acupuncture sessions covered by your insurance. Also, certain states, including California, Florida, Oregon, and Washington tend to provide better insurance coverage for acupuncture than others. If your insurance company will not cover acupuncture treatments, a Health Savings Account (HSA) could be helpful. You can use an HSA to pay for your treatments, which may lower their cost, since HSA funds often come out of your paycheck on a pre-tax basis.

OUTCOMES AND COMPLICATIONS

Acupuncture has been shown to reduce tremors from ET.[1-3] In one study, once weekly acupuncture treatments for ten weeks reduced tremors and improved writing and ease of eating and drinking for a year after the treatments ended.[1] Another study found there was a 90% decrease in tremors when they were treated with acupuncture and medicine together, compared to a 56% decrease in tremors treated with medicine alone.[4] In a study on patients with Parkinson's disease, tremors and symptoms such as slowness of movement decreased with twice weekly acupuncture treatment.[5] Acupuncture may also help your anxiety or nervousness, depression, sleep issues, and other symptoms.[6] This area of medicine has yet to be studied fully.

There are very few known side effects from acupuncture. With qualified and well-trained acupuncturists, the main issue is temporary slight bruising at the sites of needle placement. This may be related to medicines that people take. There have been other side effects reported, including infections, nerve injury, and other very rare complications including lung or heart injury, which may be caused by poor needle technique.[7] If you take care to find an acupuncturist who is licensed in your state and has received the right training, you are unlikely to have any major side effects from treatment.

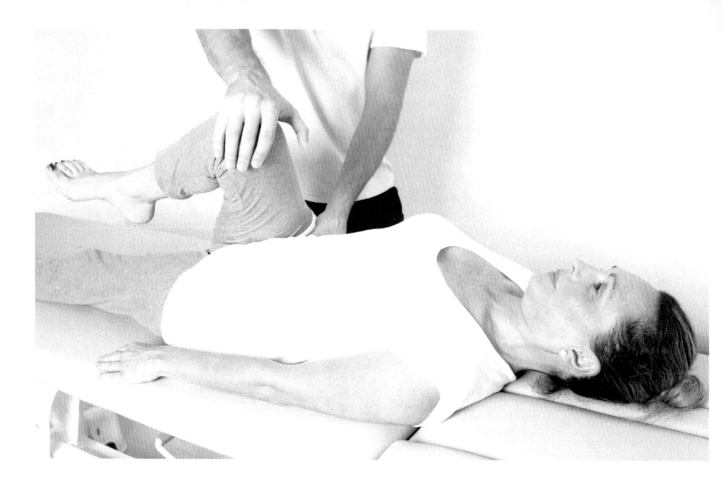

CHIROPRACTIC TREATMENT

What it is and how it works

Chiropractic treatments are procedures done by chiropractors, who are medical professionals who use their hands to manipulate (adjust) your back or neck bones, joints, or muscles. They can treat many different problems with your nerves or muscles. Often people think that chiropractors only treat back or neck pain, much like acupuncture. While this is one area they treat, chiropractors may also treat other medical problems, including tremors. We do not really understand how chiropractic treatment can help treat tremors; we simply know that it can work.

Where to find a chiropractor

A chiropractor is a licensed professional who has finished college and four years of chiropractic school. They are called doctors, as their degree is a Doctor of Chiropractic (DC), though they have not done as much training as medical doctors, who do a "residency" that lasts between three and eight years after medical school. Chiropractors are licensed by the medical board in the state in which they practice. When you find a chiropractor, you should search on the internet to check that his or her license is up to date in your state. Your general doctor also may be able to recommend a chiropractor. Like acupuncturists, chiropractors are often found in "holistic medicine" centers or centers for "integrative medicine." You can also find a chiropractor by searching the websites for the American Chiropractic Association (www.acatoday.org) or World Chiropractic Alliance (www.worldchiropracticalliance.org). It is important to ask if your chiropractor has experience in treating tremors. Not all chiropractors are trained in the adjustment procedures that treat tremors.

What to expect

Chiropractic visits may last anywhere from 15 minutes to an hour. Expect your first visit to take the longest. On your first visit with your chiropractor, he or she will ask you questions about your medical problems. Be sure to mention all of your medical problems, including medicines you take, because this may change your treatment. Also, be sure to tell your chiropractor about any pain or tingling feelings in your back, neck, arms, or legs, and mention if you think one of your arms or legs is weaker than the other. This is important, because sometimes these symptoms mean you have a problem with your spine or spinal cord. You would need to have that checked out by your regular doctor before having chiropractic treatment.

Your chiropractor will also do a physical exam, which involves pressing on the bones and muscles in your back and neck. You will also likely have x-rays taken of your neck and back to make sure you do not have other problems that need a different kind of treatment. You will then lie down on a table, and your chiropractor will use his or her hands to make quick movements that will move your bones, joints, and/or muscles. This is called an "adjustment." You may hear or feel a popping sound or sensation after an adjustment. This should not be painful. If you were having pain when you came into the office, it should get better after the adjustment.

You may also have "vibration therapy," which involves placing a small instrument on your wrist, arm, or hand in various spots for a few seconds at a time. Your chiropractor may give you stretching exercises to do and will have you come back for follow-up visits. These may be twice a week at first and may eventually be reduced to weekly and monthly visits. After each visit, it is helpful to drink a lot of water and do gentle muscle stretches to help the toxins (substances your body makes or that you are exposed to that can be harmful) get out of your system.

Outcomes and complications

There are a few reports of cases in which chiropractic treatment has improved tremors caused by Parkinson's disease[8] and ET.[9] This has not been well studied, though, so there is no proof that the improvements in these patients were due to chiropractic treatments. There are some risks to chiropractic treatment, including nerve and spinal cord damage. When a qualified chiropractor is using good techniques, the risk of these complications is very rare.

Cost and insurance coverage

The cost of each chiropractic treatment usually ranges between $50 and $150 depending on which treatments are used. This cost can vary, as with acupuncture, if you buy "packages" of several visits at a time. Your insurance company may cover a limited number of chiropractic visits. However, as with acupuncture, you will usually need to be treated for pain in order for the visit to be covered. You can also use an HSA to pay for visits to the chiropractor.

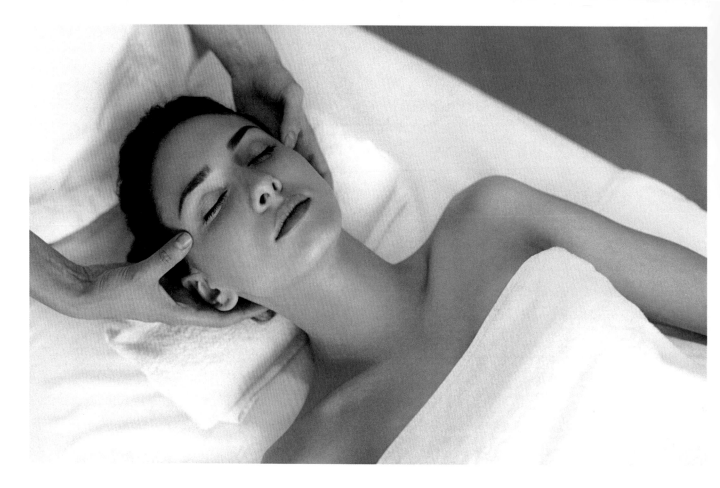

MASSAGE THERAPY

What it is

Massage therapy is a technique in which a massage therapist presses or rubs muscles in the body in order to make tight muscles relax. Massage therapy is usually done to decrease stress or ease pain from an injury. Massage therapy generally involves gentle movements, as opposed to the abrupt movements of chiropractic treatments, although deep pressure is sometimes used during massage.

How it works

Massage is thought to decrease tremors by activating certain nerves that help the body relax. There are two systems in the body that work together but sometimes compete, called the "sympathetic" and "parasympathetic" nervous systems. When one of these two systems is not working well, it can cause the other system to work abnormally too. Think of the sympathetic nervous system as the one that wants to "protect" your body from anything bad happening to it. This system is active when you are threatened by something, such as a bear running after you. In this case, your sympathetic nervous system would give you more energy in your muscles, more air in your lungs, and help your heart beat faster—all these things would give you a better chance of outrunning the bear. In the same way, when you have a disease or illness, your sympathetic nervous system senses a threat and tries to protect your body. When you have a chronic (long-term) illness such as tremor, this system does not work normally.[10]

The parasympathetic nervous system is the one that is active when you are calm. One of the effects of this system is that your muscles become relaxed. When your muscles are relaxed, your tremors decrease. Not sure about this? Think about when your tremors are worse and when they are better. They are worse when you are stressed—and when you are stressed, your muscles are usually tense. Your tremors are often better after a relaxing bath, or sometimes a glass of wine. Your muscles are more relaxed at these times. Try an experiment to see this work: Hold a five-pound weight in your hand with your arm straight out for five minutes and then put it down and try to pick up a coffee cup. Your tremors are worse, right? Well, your muscles were tight for those five minutes you were holding up the weight. Now, do some gentle stretches for five minutes to help your muscles relax. Now hold that coffee cup again. How are your tremors? Better, right? So imagine how fifty to sixty minutes of muscle relaxation during a massage could help your tremors!

Where to find a massage therapist

Massage therapists are relatively easy to find. Most cities usually have multiple massage centers. When searching online, you will want to search for a "massage center" or "massage therapy." Avoid search terms such as "massage parlor." That will lead you to a different kind of massage than that which is recommended for your tremors. As with other practitioners, massage therapists should have licenses to practice. Their licenses should be listed on your state's medical board website. The good news is, while there are a few techniques that help tremors more than others, most massage techniques that help your muscles relax will also help your tremors improve.

WHAT TO EXPECT

Most massages last from 50 minutes to an hour. You can schedule longer sessions, usually up to two hours, if desired. Expect to have a short consultation (5-10 minutes) with your massage therapist before your session. You will want to discuss all of your medical problems, and make sure you mention any recent surgeries you have had or particularly painful places on your body. Your therapist will want to use lighter pressure on those areas or avoid them altogether. After your consultation, your therapist will leave the room, and you will undress (keeping your undergarments on if you wish) and lie under a sheet on a padded table. These tables are often heated. When you are ready, your therapist will come back into the room. You can also ask for a pillow for your back or legs to make yourself more comfortable.

Your therapist will often use an oil or lotion to gently massage your back, neck, arms, legs, and sometimes your stomach or head. Only the part of your body being massaged will be uncovered. The rest of your body will stay under the sheet. About halfway through the massage, your therapist will ask you to flip over to continue the massage on the other side of your body. It is helpful during a massage to try to relax by taking deep breaths and either clearing your mind or thinking about happy things. You should tell your massage therapist during the massage if the pressure he or she is using is too hard or not hard enough, so that it can be adjusted for your comfort. Massage should not hurt! So tell your therapist right away if something he or she is doing hurts.

After the session, your therapist will usually talk to you about your session. Be sure to mention anything you liked or did not like, so that next time your therapist can change your treatment. You will want to drink a lot of water for 24 hours after your massage, because it will help get the toxins that are released during massage out of your body. You will likely be asked to schedule more massages once a week or every other week to continue helping your tremors. When you schedule follow-up appointments, it is helpful (but not crucial) to schedule your massages with the same person so you can get the most benefit out of your sessions.

There are a few studies that show massage helps reduce tremors from ET and Parkinson's disease. A recent study[11] reviewed all previous research on ways regular massage can reduce tremor. Overall, the research shows that massage can decrease shaking by 25% in some cases to almost 100% in other cases. Techniques of massage that have worked include traditional "Swedish" massage, neuromuscular therapy (involves deeper pressure), and applying heat to certain muscles during the massage.[12] Successful treatments that decrease tremors in the long term usually happen once a week.

The cost of a massage can vary greatly, from as low as $60 for an hour to over $200 for a 50-minute session. Generally, massage therapists who work at a spa or hotel are costlier. This does not necessarily mean they are better. You can often find a local massage therapist who will do a great job on the lower end of this price range. If you sign up for weekly massages, some centers will give you a discounted price. It is rare for insurance companies to cover massages, but you should ask your company to find out. You can usually pay for massages using an HSA, and if your doctor or chiropractor writes a "prescription" for the massage, then you can deduct this cost from your taxes.

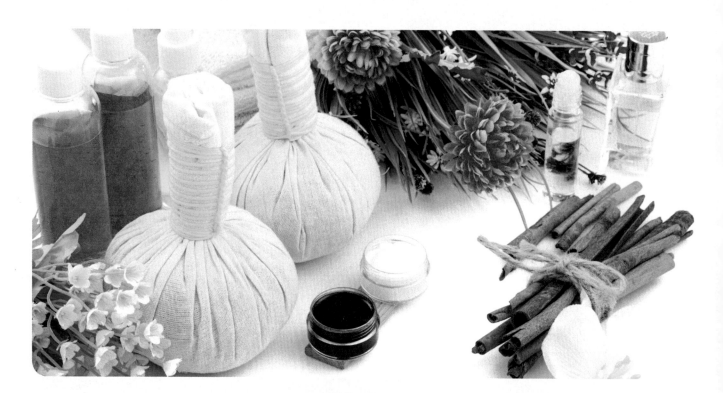

OTHER THERAPIES

There are several other alternative therapies that have been suggested to improve or eliminate tremors. These include aromatherapy, hydrotherapy, polarity therapy, and reflexology.[13] None of these have been formally researched. Most of these therapies do not have serious side effects, so they may be safe methods to try to reduce your tremors. As always, please consult with your doctor before starting any new therapy, even if it is considered "safe."

CHAPTER SUMMARY

Therapy	Frequency suggested	Benefits	Cost per treatment
Acupuncture	1x/week - 2x/month	long-term	$40-$150
Chiropractic	1x/week - 2x/month	unknown	$50-$150
Massage	1x/week	short-term	$60-$200

REFERENCES

1. Mir S, Hsiao E, Hutton MR. Acupuncture for the temporary treatment of essential tremor: a case report. *Adv Mind Body Med.* 2015;29(2):26-30.

2. Jeong JJ, Sun SH. Sa-am five-element acupuncture and hwangyeon-haedoktang pharmacopuncture treatment for an essential tremor: three case reports. *J Pharmacopuncture.* 2013;16(4):49-53.

3. de la Torre CS. Benign essential tremor resolved with acupuncture. *Medical Acupuncture. A Journal for Physicians by Physicians.* 1989;1(1).

4. Sui KM, Li X. [Clinical observation on acupuncture combined with medication for treatment of essential tremor. *Zhongguo Zhen Jiu.*] 2010;30(2):107-9. [Article in Chinese]

5. Shulman LM, Wen X, Weiner WJ, et al. Acupuncture therapy for the symptoms of Parkinson's disease. *Mov Disord.* 2002;17(4):799-802.

6. de Lorent L, Agorastos A, Yassouridis A, Kellner M, Muhtz C. Auricular acupuncture versus progressive muscle relaxation in patients with anxiety disorders or major depressive disorder a prospective parallel group clinical trial. *J Acupunct Meridian Stud.* 2016;9(4):191-9.

7. Xu S, Wang L, Cooper E, et al. Adverse events of acupuncture: a systematic review of case reports. *Evid Based Complement Alternat Med.* 2013:581203.

8. Bova J, Sergent A. Chiropractic management of an 81-year-old man with Parkinson disease signs and symptoms. *J Chiropr Med.* 2014;13(2):116-20.

9. Hubbard TA, Kane JD. Chiropractic management of essential tremor and migraine: a case report. *J Chiropr Med.* 2012;11(2):121-6.

10. Habipoglu Y, Alpua M, Bilkay C, Turkel Y, Dag E. Autonomic dysfunction in patients with essential tremor. *Neurol Sci.* 2017;38(2):265-269.

11. Casciaro Y. Massage therapy treatment and outcomes for a patient with Parkinson's disease: a case report. *Int J Ther Massage Bodywork.* 2016;9(1):11-8.

12. Riou N. Massage therapy for essential tremor: quieting the mind. *J Bodyw Mov Ther.* 2013;17(4):488-94.

13. Complementary Therapies. National Tremor Foundation website. http://tremor.org.uk/alternative-therapies.html.

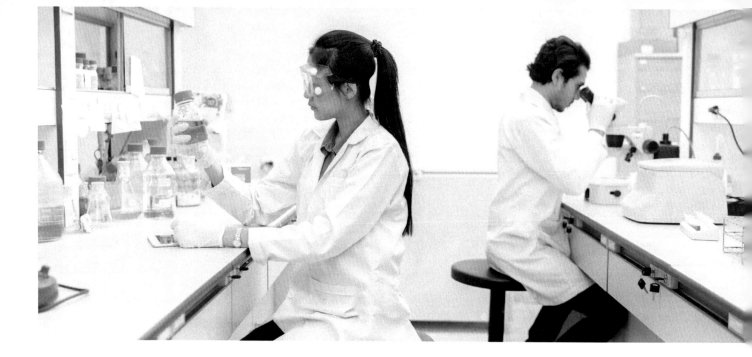

RESEARCH

Medical research helps us find new ways to treat medical problems more effectively and more safely. Because we do not fully understand what causes people with essential tremor (ET) to shake, research on it has been a little difficult. In general, when we know what causes a medical condition, we can make a research plan to find ways to either change the source of the problem or get around the problem. In the case of ET, we do not know for certain what is causing the problem. Looking for a solution to a problem we do not understand can be difficult!

Consider the following example. Imagine that your internet service went out in your house. There could be a number of possible reasons for this, such as: a circuit breaker tripped in the room where your router is, cable or phone lines are down, or you forgot to pay your bill. The problem could also be caused by things you may not even realize or that are out of your control. Maybe your dog chewed through one of the cables going to your router, or maybe your internet service provider stopped providing service to your area without sending you a notice. So there are a number of ways you can try to "troubleshoot" the cause of your problem. In fact,

you may not ever find a direct solution and may need to create a "workaround," such as using your smartphone for internet access instead.

This same process applies to medical research for conditions such as ET, in which we do not know for certain what the problem is. In ET, we believe the problem may involve chemical and/or electrical circuits in the brain. So research studies currently focus on these areas. Below are studies that, at the time of the writing of this book in early 2018, either are in progress or have recently completed testing in patients. These are not yet considered "standard" therapies for the treatment of tremor. As new findings become public, I will be updating this book's website (www.helpfortremors.com) with information about these results and about other new research studies.

IMPORTANT NOTE: Treatments presented in this section of the book are not yet available to the public, so your doctor may not be able to refer you for one of these treatments.

Transcranial magnetic stimulation (TMS) is a treatment that involves using magnets placed near a person's head to control tremors and a number of other medical problems (e.g., depression, pain, etc.). TMS is thought to work by changing the way brain cells communicate with each other, and it can change both electrical and chemical activity in the brain. Studies have tried placing the magnets in different spots near the top and back of the head to see what the effects are. Some of these studies have found that tremors caused by ET or Parkinson's disease can be decreased with a single TMS treatment, while other studies suggest that several treatments within the span of a week to a few weeks are needed to see improvements.[1] So, while this treatment can be helpful, it is not yet clear how to best use this treatment to control tremors.[2] There is a current study on this treatment being done in Iran that is expected to end in February 2018 and another study in France that is expected to finish in May 2018.

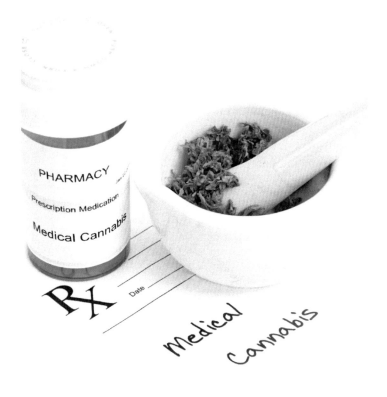

OCTANOIC ACID

Octanoic acid (OA) is a medicine that can be given in pill form to patients with tremor to control their shaking. OA is a type of alcohol that does not give you the same side effects as you would have drinking wine, beer, or liquor. Just as alcohol that you drink can help your tremor, studies have shown that OA can help decrease tremors. However, the problem is that the dose (amount) of OA needed to control tremors is very high, which means it is hard to get the right amount of medicine in a single or even many pills. Also, side effects from these very high doses include sleepiness,[3] belly pain, and diarrhea.[4] OA is currently approved by the FDA for use as a "food additive" to add flavor to food; however, it is not currently approved as a treatment for ET. It is possible to change your diet to include more foods containing OA, and this is described in <u>Section 2</u> of this book.

MARIJUANA

Cannabis, also known as marijuana, is most widely known in the US as a recreational drug. However, it has many properties that can help treat certain medical conditions. One of the most popular is a chemical in cannabis called "cannabidiol" that is used in the treatment of seizures.[5] Many of the medicines used to treat tremors caused by ET are medicines made to treat seizures (e.g., Primidone, Gabapentin, Topiramate), so cannabidiol has been suggested as a way to decrease tremors. Because marijuana and its related drugs have recently become fully legal in eight states in the US, and legal for medical use in another 22 states,[6] there will likely be more research coming out to study the benefits of marijuana for tremors. Currently, a few studies[7] have shown that marijuana decreases tremors caused by Parkinson's disease and multiple sclerosis. There are currently no published studies on the effects of cannabis on people with ET. However, some studies in animals have shown that medicines made with cannabis-like chemicals may improve tremor.[8]

One theory about the cause of essential tremor involves a chemical made in the brain called GABA. Studies have shown that in the brains of ET patients, there is not as much GABA as in an average person's brain, or GABA does not work the way that it should.[9] Some researchers[9] believe that giving baclofen, a medicine that increases GABA in the body, to people with ET will decrease their tremors. This idea is based on studies in rats[10] in which baclofen decreased tremor.

"SMART" DBS

For those who have deep brain stimulation (DBS) systems already implanted in their brains to treat their tremors, there is ongoing research looking for ways to help those systems work better. This idea is known as a "Smart" DBS system. It is also sometimes called "Responsive" or "Closed-loop" DBS. Right now, DBS systems send constant electrical pulses to the brain. Some researchers believe that if the systems could send electricals pulses only when needed ("responsive" to people's needs), people would have better tremor control and fewer side effects from DBS. The problem is in figuring out how a responsive system would know when the brain needs stimulation. Some studies suggest that when an amount of a certain chemical or chemicals in the brain is low, this should trigger an electrical pulse.[11] Other researchers believe a change in electrical activity in the brain should be the trigger for the pulse.[12] Early results from all these studies have shown very positive results.[13]

New studies are being developed on a regular basis. For the most up-to-date information, visit www.clinicaltrials.gov and search for studies related to ET or other conditions. You can narrow your search to "Currently Recruiting" to see what trials may be available in your area. At the time of the writing of this book, there were 33 currently recruiting studies worldwide that are studying ways to improve the diagnosis or treatment of ET. If you are interested in learning more about a study, you can contact the researchers, or "investigators," directly. Each study on the website has contact information with a phone number and/or email listed.

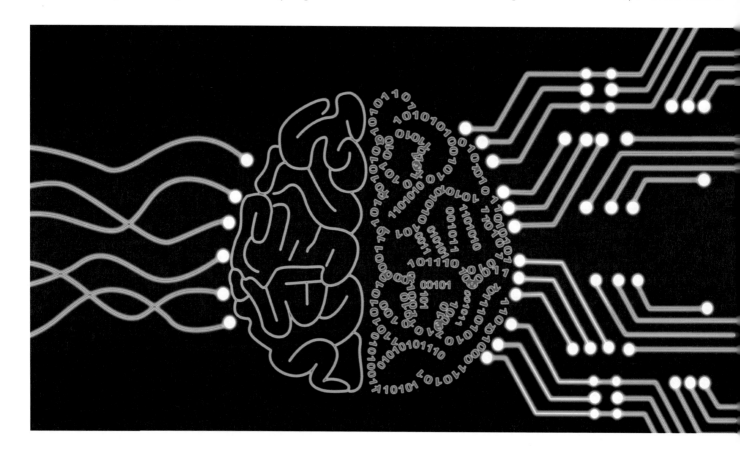

REFERENCES

1. Shih LC, Pascual-Leone A. Non-invasive brain stimulation for essential tremor. *Tremor Other Hyperkinet Mov (N Y)*. 2017;7:458.

2. Obeso I, Cerasa A, Quattrone A. The effectiveness of transcranial brain stimulation in improving clinical signs of hyperkinetic movement disorders. *Front Neurosci*. 2016;9:486.

3. Voller B, Lines E, McCrossin G, et al. Dose-escalation study of octanoic acid in patients with essential tremor. *J Clin Invest*. 2016;126(4):1451-7.

4. Haubenberger D, Nahab FB, Voller B, Hallett M. Treatment of essential tremor with long-chain alcohols: still experimental or ready for prime time? *Tremor Other Hyperkinet Mov (N Y)*. 2014;4:tre-04-222-4763-2.

5. Perucca E. Cannabinoids in the treatment of epilepsy: hard evidence at last? *J Epilepsy Res*. 2017;7(2):61-76.

6. State Marijuana Laws 2018 Map. Governing website. http://www.governing.com/gov-data/state-marijuana-laws-map-medical-recreational.html. January 8, 2018.

7. Kluger B, Triolo P, Jones W, Jankovic, J. The therapeutic potential of cannabinoids for movement disorders. *Mov Disord*. 2015;30(3):313–327.

8. Abbassian H, Whalley BJ, Sheibani V, Shabani M. Cannabinoid type 1 receptor antagonism ameliorates harmaline-induced essential tremor in rat. *Br J Pharmacol*. 2016;173(22):3196–3207.

9. Hamad M, Holland R, Kamal N, Luceri R, Mammis A. Potential for Intrathecal Baclofen in Treatment of Essential Tremor. *World Neurosurg*. 2017;105:170-175.

10. Tariq M, Arshaduddin M, Biary N, Al Moutaery K, Al Deeb S. Baclofen attenuates harmaline induced tremors in rats. *Neurosci Lett*. 2001;312(2):79-82.

11. Da Cunha C, Boschen SL, Gómez-A A, et al. Toward sophisticated basal ganglia neuromodulation: review on basal ganglia deep brain stimulation. *Neurosci Biobehav Rev*. 2015;58:186–210.

12. Little S, Tripoliti E, Beudel M, et al. Adaptive deep brain stimulation for Parkinson's disease demonstrates reduced speech side effects compared to conventional stimulation in the acute setting. *J Neurol Neurosurg Psychiatr*. 2016;87:1388–1389.

13. Ramirez-Zamora A, Giordano JJ, Gunduz A, et al. Evolving applications, technological challenges and future opportunities in neuromodulation: proceedings of the fifth annual deep brain stimulation think tank. *Front Neurosci*. 2017;11:734.

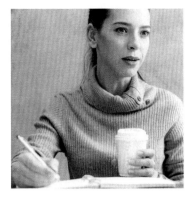
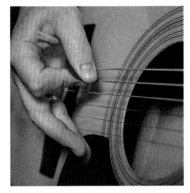
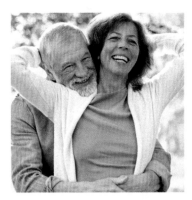
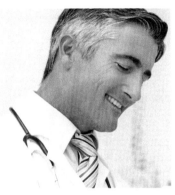
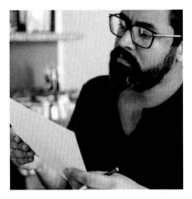
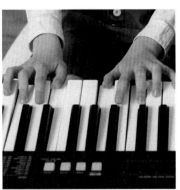
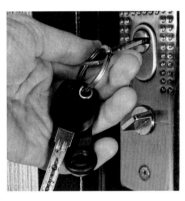
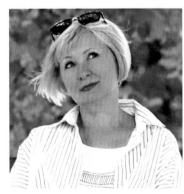
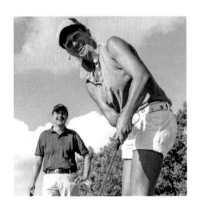

SECTION

5

**CHOOSING THE
TREATMENT THAT
IS RIGHT FOR YOU**

CHOOSING TREATMENT
THAT IS RIGHT FOR YOU

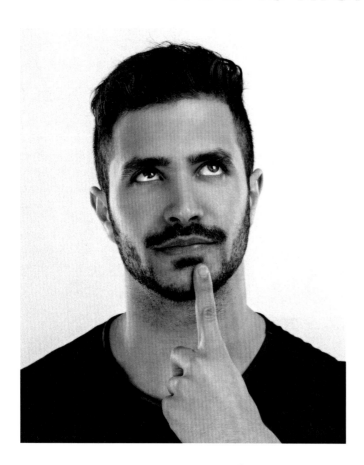

Choices are everywhere! It seems like every time we turn around, we are faced with yet another decision! And choices in medical care can be even more overwhelming. If you make the wrong choice, it is possible bad things could happen. You could get sicker. You could even die. This is scary stuff! So, often you rely on your doctor to tell you what he or she recommends, because you trust your doctor will do what is best for you, keep you safe, and offer solutions that heal and do not harm. That takes a lot of pressure off of you, right?

Yet somehow, handing the power of choice over to someone else, no matter how knowledgeable, can feel frightening, too. A recent study showed that most essential tremor (ET) patients actually want more treatment choices and more control in deciding what their treatment will be.[1] Are you among

those people who want more control over their choices? Even if you are not and would rather have your doctor decide for you, sometimes your doctor will give you more than one recommendation and ask you to choose. Yikes! Now what? Now the choice is back in your hands, and you once again feel the weight of the decision on your shoulders.

As I have told you a few times before in this book, please take a moment and breathe. Relax. It is going to be okay. I am here to help you learn how to make choices for your health. And with this knowledge, you will feel empowered, gain confidence, and find peace in your decisions—much more peace than you would have if you were to let someone else make your choices for you.

THE SCIENCE OF CHOICE

First, let us take a moment to understand what is going on in your brain when you try to make a decision. This very much depends on your state of mind: your brain thinks very differently when you are making a decision "in the moment" and with a lot of emotion than when you have plenty of time to decide.

The effect of stress on your brain

Making decisions when emotions are high causes a stress reaction in your brain. As described earlier in this book, stress causes two major changes in your body. First, your body goes into "fight or flight" mode and activates your "sympathetic nervous system." This is the system that wants to "protect" you from bad things happening. Your brain starts to "think" with its protective part, the brainstem, whose main goal is to keep you breathing and keep your heart beating. Your brain stops relying on other, more rational areas that can weigh your choices and think about the long-term consequences of your decisions. In this stress state, your brain starts looking for the quickest available solution, so it overlooks other choices that may be better for you. The sympathetic nervous system does not work "normally" in people with chronic illnesses,[2] so if you have a condition such as ET or Parkinson's disease, you could have even more difficulty making decisions under stress.

Second, your body releases a stress hormone called cortisol, which then causes an increase in another chemical in your brain called dopamine.[3] When your dopamine levels are high, this can give you a feeling of euphoria or extreme happiness. You may focus more on the good things that could happen, such as the benefits of a treatment, rather than the bad things, such as the risks. So, if you feel pressured to make a decision quickly, or if you are really worried about your medical condition, you may end up choosing the first treatment presented to you or one that is risky.

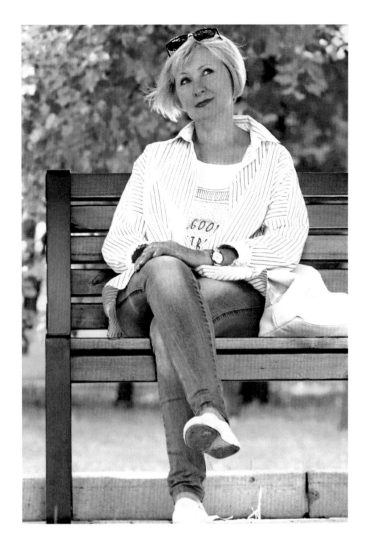

Gender and age-related effects

There are a couple of other things that affect how we make choices under stress. These are related to whether you are a man or a woman and to how old you are. In stressful situations, women tend to take fewer risks, while men tend to take more.[3] In regular, non-stressful situations, this difference between men and women does not occur. Further, when under stress, older people tend to prefer more "certain" choices, while younger people are willing to take greater risks for a better result. For instance, an older person may choose a therapy that has helped 90 out of 100 people make their tremors at least 50 percent better. A younger person, on the other hand, may prefer a treatment that has a 50/50 chance of working but could make their tremors 99 percent better.[4]

Calming down your brain

When you are calmer, less emotionally driven, and not under a time limit, your brain tends to think with a more rational area that is able to analyze complex problems. In this state, your brain will carefully weigh all the risks and benefits of a decision and then make a choice based on facts. This is how you want your brain to think whenever possible. So, how do you get it there if you are really worried about a decision?

There are a few tricks you can use to calm your brain down so you can make well thought-out, rational choices that will most benefit you in the long term. First, before you start to make any decision, I encourage you to take a moment and do a short meditation and visualization exercise. You can refer to the techniques described in Section 2 to help you do this. Taking time to settle your mind into a positive state is probably the most helpful thing you can do before you start to make a decision. If you are anxious about making a decision, these techniques will also help you decrease your anxiety. They help counteract the brain's natural stress response, allowing the parts of your brain that are great at analyzing complex problems to take over. Meditation and visualization can help you any time you need to make a decision, even when you do not feel stressed.

Another trick is to ask yourself, or have someone else ask you, a question that needs at least two steps to answer. This question does not have to be related to what is causing you stress. In fact, it is often better if it is not related. The simple act of asking yourself this question does a couple of things. First, it distracts your brain from the current stressful situation. Second, because it requires careful thought, the question makes your brain "wake up" and respond. Once the rational part of your brain starts thinking through a problem, you will be in a much better position to think about a solution to something that causes you stress and anxiety.

For example, when I am feeling overwhelmed, I may stop and ask myself something like this: "I wonder who is going to win the Masters Golf Tournament next month?" First, I have to stop and remember who is invited to the tournament, and then I have think through how well each golfer has been playing this year. I do not have to actually settle on an answer; I simply need to make my brain start thinking through a problem. In addition to helping calm your brain before making medical decisions, this technique will put you in a calmer, more rational state of mind any time you are in an emotionally charged situation.

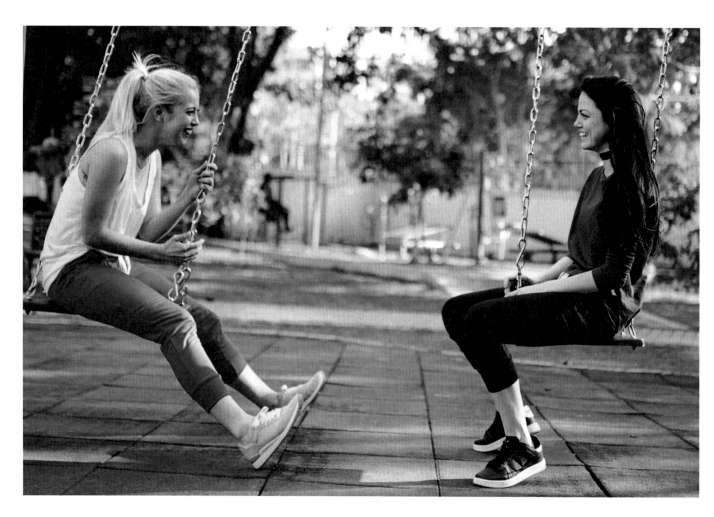

Now that you understand what is going on in your brain when you are trying to make a decision, I will introduce you to a method that I have coached thousands of people to use when thinking through decisions. As I doctor, I have guided people through decisions that were minor, such as choosing one medicine over another, as well as major, such as deciding whether to take a family member off of life support. I also use this method when making decisions for myself. It is certainly not the only way to work through decisions about your medical care, but I hope this helps make the process a little bit easier.

IDEAL SCENARIO

First, I ask you to envision your ideal scenario as it relates to your tremor. You may think, "Well, my ideal scenario is that I have nothing wrong with me!" That is exactly what I want you to think about. Think about your life with no tremor. Think about the things you want to be able to do—the things that are most important to you. Do you want to go back to work? Do you want to enjoy golf again? Do you want to spend more time with your grandchildren? Take time to write this out or think it through. The most important part of medical decision making is to know why you want to feel better. Knowing this will be a critical part of both making choices and following through with the choices you make.

Now, look at your list of goals and make sure it is complete. Have you left anything off? **Do not negotiate with yourself.** Maybe you will not get to do everything on your list, but maybe you will. Write down every goal you have for your life without tremor, even ones that seem impossible to accomplish. Then, rank your goals in order of importance. What is the most important thing you want to be able to do without tremor? Did you write down "go back to work" because you thought you "should" write it first? Would you actually rather be able to make your lunch and eat it without spilling everything all over the kitchen? Or would being able to write letters and sign your name legibly be the one thing that brings you the most happiness? Whatever that is for you, list it at the top. This is your number one goal.

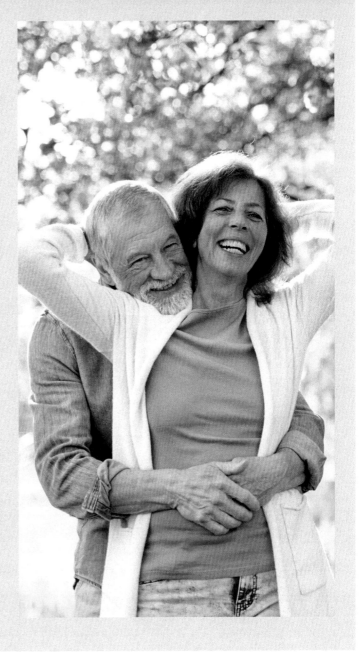

Understand the big picture regarding treatment choices

Now that you have a clear idea in your mind of what you want, you need to understand the big picture regarding your treatment choices. What do I mean by this? Start by making broad categories of your options. Is taking medicine a choice for treatment? What about surgery or alternative medicine? Are there diet and exercise changes you can make? Remember that "doing nothing" is also a choice—one that often has consequences. Write that down as one of your categories. Resist the urge to "judge" these options right now. Do not worry about whether you think they will or will not work. Just write the categories down.

Understand the different options in each category

Now that you have a list of a few general treatment categories, you can fill in specific options under each one. How many medicines could possibly treat your condition? Two? Write down the names of both of them. How many surgery options are there? Four? Write those down as well. How many different diets and exercise choices are there? What about alternative therapies? Fill in the names of all your options under each category.

Get the facts about each option

Start with one general category and learn the facts about each option in that category. For example, if you start with medicine, learn about each medicine you wrote down. How well does it work? Does it work for everyone? How much better can it make your tremor? What are the risks of taking it? How long will it take to work? How much does it cost?

Be careful where you get your information! You will not help yourself if your only source of information about these treatments is from a chat room on the internet or a group post on social media. Sometimes people with unusual conditions or rare reactions to a treatment will post about them online more than people who have no issues with a treatment. This can give you a warped idea of how common a particular side effect or complication is. The highest quality information you will get is from your medical doctors and from reputable books, books, and certain websites that back up information with medical research.

> NOTE: Your doctor may have told you that one of these treatments is not a choice for you. For example, say you have asthma, and your doctor has already told you that you cannot take beta blockers like propranolol. You may want to cross that choice off your list now instead of taking time to learn facts about it, since it will not be an option for you.

Compare your options to your ideal scenario

Next, look at all the information you have and compare it to your ideal scenario. Think about the best and worst possible outcomes of each treatment and see how those would affect your most important goals. For example, if you take propranolol for tremor, the best outcome is that you are among the 50 percent of people for whom this medicine works, and your tremor will be reduced by half. The medicine usually works fairly quickly, so it should reduce your tremor within a week or two. And your insurance will cover the cost of the medicine, so it will only cost you five dollars per month. The worst outcome with propranolol is that you are among the 50 percent of people for whom it does not work at all. You are also one of the people who gets several side effects, so you will be tired and dizzy and depressed as long as you are taking the medicine. Your insurance will not cover the cost of the medicine, so you will also be out 50 dollars each month.

Now, say your number one goal is to be able to write letters legibly, and your tremor is moderate from the start. Then in the best-case scenario, you will have a good chance of reaching your goal in two weeks, with little to lose other than five dollars each month. Take a moment and think about how that makes you feel. How would you rate your happiness on a scale from 1 to 10 if you could accomplish your most important goal within two weeks and have it only cost you five dollars?

What if the worst possible outcome happens instead? Then you will be right where you were before you took the medicine—still unable to write letters, but you also have side effects (that likely will go away when you stop the medicine) and are out 50 dollars. Think about how this scenario makes you feel. On a scale from 1 to 10, how annoyed or scared are you by this possibility? Would you wish you had never tried it? Would this failure make you want to give up hope? Or would you still be glad you tried it and move on to try another option?

If your number one goal instead is to go back to work as a policeman, then the best- and worst-case scenarios for this treatment choice would affect you very differently. A medicine that improves your tremor by only 50 percent may not be good enough to help you get back to work. Also, the side effects could make it very difficult for you to do your job.

Use this same thought process for each treatment choice in each category. Think carefully about how you feel in the best- and worst-case scenarios. I like using a number scale from 1 to 10 as a rating, because it gives me an easy way to compare how I feel about different treatments. This becomes important when it is time to start narrowing down choices.

If there are many different treatment options for your condition, as there are for tremor, then do not feel like you have to write out all of this in one sitting! Take your time. Tremor is one medical condition that, in most cases, allows you the luxury of time to make your treatment decisions.

NARROWING DOWN YOUR CHOICES

Now that you have thought through all your options, it is time to start narrowing them down. Do not let this overwhelm you. There is a simple, logical way to do this that I find works for almost everyone. Rather than picking the best out of 25 options, you will start by eliminating choices. As you did when gathering information about the different options, you will start with the broad categories first.

The first thing I want you to do is to eliminate any category (e.g., medicine, surgery, exercise, etc.) that you do not feel comfortable doing now that you know more about it. If there is truly not one option in that category you would consider, just put a big "x" through the whole category. You may have different reasons for wanting to eliminate one whole category. For example, if you do not even want to think about being responsible for taking another medicine every day, in addition to what you already take, then eliminate the "medicine" category as a choice. Or, if it is really important to you that a lot of medical research has been done on a treatment before you are willing to try it, even if it is low risk, then the "exercise" category would be off your list.

Next, look at your remaining categories, go through the individual options under each one, and follow the same elimination process. For example, after reading about the risks of deep brain stimulation and considering the worst-case scenario, you decide you would never consider that surgery. So, cross this option off your list. Further, if the best outcome of a treatment will not help you achieve your number goal, then eliminate that option as well. For example, if you want to return to playing second string violin in your city's orchestra, and you have a fairly noticeable tremor, then any treatment choice that will only cut your tremor in half should be crossed off your list. You likely will need a treatment that can reduce your tremor by 80 percent or more.

Again, do not negotiate with yourself. I have had patients tell me that they would not ever want to have surgery, yet they wind up in my office. If something is "off the table" for you, then do not let it become a choice! One word of caution here: only make this decision once you understand all the facts. If you have decided you would never want surgery because "something bad" has happened to every person you know who has ever had surgery, or because you read horror stories on the internet, get the facts first and understand what the risks truly are.

Finalizing your choices

By now, most people will have only a few choices left. If you still have more than five choices at this point, I recommend you spend another few minutes systematically going through them again. Eliminate any treatment option that you think only has a small chance of helping you reach your top goals.

Now it is time to start looking at your options in a different way. So far, you have been eliminating choices based on what does NOT match with your goals— in terms of either the benefits of a treatment not being enough, or the risks of a treatment being too high. Now you will instead select the one or more options that best suit your goals.

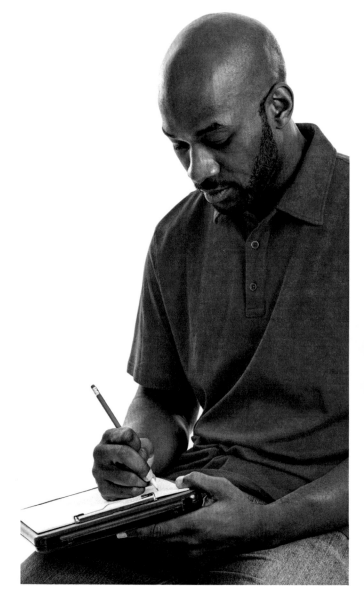

At this point, I like to make a notecard for each choice—you can write out the name of each treatment or use a picture. Use whatever format will be easiest for you to identify the treatments. On each notecard, you may want to write down the benefit or risk of that treatment that stands out to you the most. You may also want to write down the number (between 1 and 10) you associated with the best outcome and the number you associated with the worst outcome. Then, lay all of these notecards out in front of you.

Take a moment to adjust your frame of mind

Before you do anything else, I recommend you take a moment and put yourself in a positive mindset, as you hopefully did before you started this exercise. Take five minutes and remind yourself about the goals that you have and the things you want to be able to do. Visualize yourself doing these things (see "The Power of Visualization" in <u>Section 2</u>). Now you are in a much better position to look at the choices you have left and to make the decision that will get you closest to your goals.

Next, think about the following treatment outcomes and rank how important they are in relation to your top goal:

- *Minimal or no tremor*
- *No or low risk*
- *Fast results*
- *Low cost*

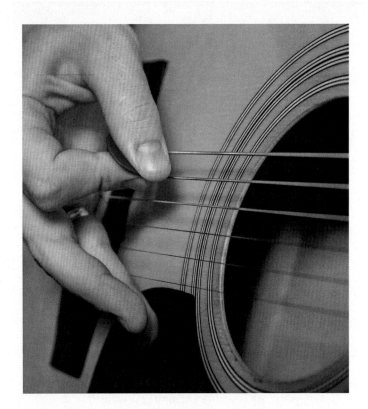

Returning to our example, say your goal is to be able to write letters legibly. Perhaps having a safe treatment is most important to you, even more than having no tremor. Then "no or low risk" goes at the top of your ranking, followed by "minimal or no tremor." Maybe how long it takes for the treatment to work is not important to you, so "fast results" goes at the bottom of your ranking. Finally, perhaps you are not too concerned about the price of treatment, so "low cost" comes third in your ranking.

Now, look at the notecards with your treatment choices. Choose the one or two treatments that match best your top goal. Staying with our example, say you have tried medicines already, and those have not worked. After going through all the steps above and narrowing down your treatment options, you are left with the following: deep brain stimulation, Gamma Knife, focused ultrasound, a research study, and the Mediterranean diet. As "no or low risk" is your top priority, you would now select focused ultrasound and Mediterranean diet as your top two possibilities. Since your second most important priority is "minimal or no tremor," you would then choose focused ultrasound.

If, after you have completed the whole process, you still have more than one treatment choice on your list, then you should go with your "gut instinct." Only do this when you have already done all of the preceding steps. Otherwise, you will be making a decision without logically and carefully considering all of the facts.

Keep in mind two things. First, some treatment options will require that you try another treatment first. As mentioned in the chapter on "Surgical Treatment," you will not be offered any surgical procedure without first trying to control your tremor with medicine. Second, you can often try more than one treatment option at the same time. Your goal is to reduce your tremor, not to perform a scientific experiment to see how successful any one treatment is. So, as long as your doctor has said it is safe, you can consider trying multiple ways to reduce your tremor. Please note that if you develop side effects while using multiple methods to treat your tremor, it may be difficult to tell which treatment is causing the side effects. You can either eliminate one treatment at a time to figure this out or stop all but one treatment and slowly add others back in.

Rating your decision

Once you have made your decision about which treatment(s) to pursue, this next step is important. Think about how good you feel about your decision. How confident are you that you have made the right choice? Again, use the 1 to 10 rating scale. For me, if I rate my confidence as less than a 10, I do not settle for my choice. I think about what I would need in order to feel 100 percent confident. Usually, it is more information. So, I go back and get more information about my choices and go through the process again. The degree of confidence you want may be different than this. Some people are happy being 80 percent sure (an "8" on the rating scale) that they have made the right choice. That is completely okay! Just decide what number is enough for you and keep thinking through your decision until you get there.

Sticking with your decision

Once you are confident with your decision, you need to stick with it. Believe in your choice. If you do not fully believe that you made the right choice, then your chosen treatment may not work for you. You may be less likely, for example, to do everything exactly as you are instructed for your treatment. When you believe in your choice, you follow through. You take your medicines as the doctor orders. You follow every single pre-operative and post-operative instruction your doctor gives you. And when you do this, you have the best chance at a successful outcome, which is the outcome you envisioned in your ideal scenario.

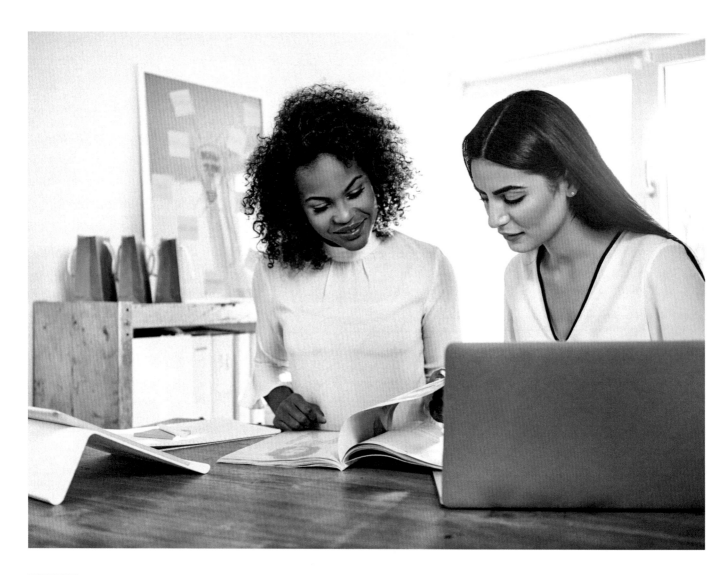

SPECIAL CIRCUMSTANCES

There are a couple of special circumstances that may require you to change the way you make decisions: when you are making a choice for someone else and when you are making a choice in an emergency situation. Often these two circumstances happen together, such as when a family member is in a car accident or has a stroke.

In these cases, emotions are heightened. As explained above, your brain is not able to process thoughts in a logical, rational way when emotions are involved. Additionally, in an emergency situation, no one wants to take the time to work through the detailed process I just described. So, making a choice for a family member and/or in an emergency situation requires a different approach.

For these situations, I often recommend what is called a "values-based approach" to decision making. This approach requires you to know and understand what you, or the person for whom you are making the decision, most value in life. Some people have a good understanding of what they most value. For me, my main values are faith, family, integrity, and perseverance. Other people value different things more highly, such as intelligence, a particular skill or talent, or financial stability. It does not matter what you most value, as long as you know what it is.

If you do not know your values off the top of your head, I encourage you to take a moment to think about them. There are also online assessments you can take to help you determine what those are, if you are having difficulty figuring them out. In an emergency situation, it is easier to start making decisions if

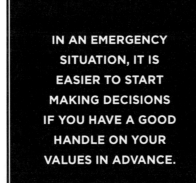

IN AN EMERGENCY SITUATION, IT IS EASIER TO START MAKING DECISIONS IF YOU HAVE A GOOD HANDLE ON YOUR VALUES IN ADVANCE.

you have a good handle on your values in advance. If you must make a quick decision for a family member whose values you do not know, you can think about what your family member spends most of his or her time doing. Is it working at a job? Or spending time with grandchildren? What about doing hobbies? Going shopping? Going to church? Thinking about this can give you a good idea about a person's values if you have never had that discussion with him or her.

Once you understand the values that are most important to someone, you can make decisions quickly. For example, if your father is an avid outdoorsman and spends most of his time hiking and fishing, then he would likely be unhappy if he could no longer do those things. So, you may choose a treatment for him that does not have as good a chance of completely fixing his medical problem but has very little risk to it. If you were to choose something that, for example, has a high risk of leaving him paralyzed, he could end up very unhappy in life.

When making choices for others in an emergency situation, it is also important that you put aside (as much as is possible) what YOU would want if you were in that situation. Everyone is different. Just because you would never have surgery does not mean your husband or your daughter would not want surgery. Keeping this in mind also helps to control the guilt you could feel if you make a decision that does not turn out well for your family member.

And remember, if you are really unsure what values are most important to your loved one, then just do your best in the moment. Know that your loved one will likely understand that you made the best decision you could. Release your guilt for anything that could happen as a result of your choice. As hard as we may try, we are not truly the One ultimately in control of the outcome.

THE POWER OF AND

I want to leave you with one final thought as I close this book. I have told you a couple of times in this last section to not "negotiate with yourself." Sometimes it seems like we cannot have everything we want. As you have read through this book, you have probably noticed that treatments with a good chance of reducing your tremors also come with a lot of risks and possible side effects. It may seem that you can choose either a treatment that will work well or a treatment that has low risk, but not both.

Many times, at first glance, it does appear that we must make choices between things and that we cannot "eat our cake and have it, too." We limit what we believe is possible because we have been taught to do so. We are taught not to ask for too much, because it only leads to disappointment. To me, this is what a life lived in fear looks like. I lived like this for a number of years. I was told that making a choice to go to medical school and become a neurosurgeon meant two things: (1) I would never have a happy family life, and (2) I would never be able to do anything else with my life, because my skill set would be too specific.

Over the past couple of years, I have come to open my mind up to the "power of AND." Sometimes, when we believe we have to make a choice, this belief is based on the limits we have placed on ourselves—limits that may not be based in reality. When we open

our minds to possibilities and let our imaginations be free to explore new ideas and concepts, we sometimes find that what we thought were limits are not in fact limits at all. The only thing we need to do is to change our perspectives and perhaps our definitions.

I have learned that it is possible to have a career as a neurosurgeon AND have a happy family life—I now have both. I have also learned that the skills I gained in the 20 years I was in training and practice as a neurosurgeon can be used to perform surgery AND in limitless other ways. My definitions and preconceived notions of what it means to be a neurosurgeon have changed. My definition of how to build a happy family has changed. And my understanding of my skill set has broadened dramatically.

I am telling you this to show you that sometimes you do not have to choose. Just because you have been told two things are not possible at the same time does not mean that is true. Let your mind have time to dream and to imagine the life you truly want. Consider not just what you have been told—consider all possibilities. I have poured all of my knowledge into this book, from the best of what I learned in my practice to the best of what other brilliant doctors and researchers have discovered. I have done this to help open your mind up to the possibilities for treating your tremor. What you choose to do with this information is up to you.

AS YOU MAKE YOUR DECISIONS, LET ME SHARE THIS WITH YOU:

I believe in a world in which people can achieve excellent tremor control AND do so with treatments that have little risk. I think the solution looks different for each and every person. I think it involves testing out different options one at a time to make sure you do not have side effects and then combining those options until your tremor is barely noticeable. For some of you, the solution could include a type of surgery or some treatment that is yet undiscovered. For many of you who try the non-surgical treatments described in this book, you may find that little by little, day by day, your tremor gets better. I do not know of one magic combination of treatments that will help everybody. I wish I did! What I do know is that the "power of AND" is strong. I was willing to give it a try. Are you?

REFERENCES

1. Louis ED, Rohl B, Rice C. Defining the treatment gap: what essential tremor patients want that they are not getting. *Tremor Other Hyperkinet Mov (N Y)*. 2015;5:331.

2. Habipoglu Y, Alpua M, Bilkay C, Turkel Y, Dag E. Autonomic dysfunction in patients with essential tremor. *Neurol Sci*. 2017;38(2):265-269.

3. Mather M, Lighthall NR. Both risk and reward are processed differently in decisions made under stress. *Curr Dir Psychol Sci*. 2012;21(2):36–41.

4. Mather M, Mazar N, Gorlick M, et al. Risk preferences and aging: the "Certainty Effect" in older adults' decision making. *Psychol Aging*. 2012;27(4):801–816.

GLOSSARY

Academic medical center — *A large hospital usually associated with a medical school or university that offers appointments with many different kinds of doctors in the same place.*

Action tremor — *Shaking that happens when a person is trying to do a specific activity, like eating, drinking, or writing. Also known as "intention tremor".*

Acupuncture — *A treatment that involves inserting tiny, thin needles into specific places in the body in order to treat illness or relieve pain.*

Activities of daily living (ADL) — *Things a person needs to do in daily life, such as eat and drink, get dressed, and take a shower or bath.*

Adaptive dressing aids — *Tools that can help people with tremor get dressed more easily.*

Adaptive tools — *Everyday products that are modified for people with tremor or other movement issues.*

Adjustment (chiropractor) — *A common chiropractic treatment that involves using the hands to make quick movements that move bones, joints, and/or muscles.*

Allergy (Medical) — *A problem that can happen after taking a medicine. This does not refer to seasonal allergies (due to pollen, dust, pet hair). Can include headache, hives, rashes, trouble breathing, swelling of the body or tongue, throwing up, or belly pain.*

Alprazolam — *A medicine used to help anxiety that can also help control tremors. A common name for this medicine is Xanax.*

Alzheimer's disease — *A type of **dementia** that causes memory loss, thinking problems, and behavior issues and gets worse over time.*

Anesthesiologist — *A doctor who gives special medicine to people going into surgery that helps them relax and feel less pain, or put them to sleep.*

Anxiety — *A condition in which a person feels constant severe nervousness or worry for a few months or more.*

Assistive devices — *Tools that can help people overcome or cope with tremor.*

Asthma — *A medical condition that causes difficulty breathing, coughing, and wheezing.*

Baclofen — *A medicine that increases the amount of **GABA** in the body and is used to help muscles relax.*

Benign essential tremor — *An older term to describe "**essential tremor**".*

Beta blocker — *A medicine that can lower blood pressure or treat heart problems after a heart attack. Can also help reduce tremor.*

Blood clot — *A clump of blood that thickens and can block an artery or a vein from carrying blood through the body.*

Blood sugar — *The amount of sugar in your blood. Also called "blood glucose". This is measured by a blood test*

Blood thinner	*A medicine that makes the blood thin. Includes Coumadin, Plavix, Eliquis, along with Aspirin, Motrin, ibuprofen, and many other over-the-counter pain medicines.*
Botox	*A medicine that is injected into a muscle to keep it from moving. Can help reduce some types of tremor. Also known as botulinum toxin.*
Brain tumor	*A mass that forms in the brain because either brain cells do not grow normally or because a cancer somewhere else in the body has spread.*
Bright light therapy	*A treatment that gives off artificial light from a box. A treatment for* **depression.** *May also improve tremor.*
Caffeine	*A substance that makes people more alert and is found in coffee, some teas and soft drinks, energy drinks, and foods such as chocolate.*
Cannabidiol	*A chemical in* **marijuana** *that is used to treat seizures.*
Cannabis	*see* **marijuana**
Caprylic acid	*see* **octanoic acid**
Carbamazepine	*A medicine used to stop seizures that can also help control tremors. A common name for this medicine is Tegretol.*
Cerebellum	*An area near the back of the brain that helps the muscles work together to create smooth movements.*
Catheter	*A tube that is inserted into the bladder to drain urine from the body.*
Chiropractor	*A medical professional who uses his/her hands to move and shift (adjust) back or neck bones, joints, or muscles.*
Chronic bronchitis	*A type of* **COPD** *that causes coughing and difficulty breathing.*
Cranial nerves	*Nerves from the base of the brain that control the ability to move the eyes, face, and head and to feel, taste, smell, see, and hear.*
Cognitive problems	*Issues that cause a person to have trouble planning and thinking normally.*
Co-pay	*The amount of money an insurance company makes people pay for doctor's appointments, medicines, and surgeries.*
COPD	*Chronic obstructive pulmonary disorder. A disease in the lungs that makes it hard to breathe. Includes chronic bronchitis and emphysema.*
Cortisol	*A chemical the body releases when a person feels stress. This chemical affects your blood sugar*
CT scan	*A special type of* **X-ray** *that takes pictures from different angles of the inside of the body. Most helpful to see bones and areas of new bleeding.*
DBS	*see* **deep brain stimulation**
Deductible	*The amount of money some insurance companies make people pay each year before their appointments, surgeries, or medicines will be covered.*
Deep brain stimulation (DBS)	*A surgery to control tremor that involves placing tiny wires with metal contacts deep inside the brain. Pulses of electricity are sent through the wires to an area of the brain that controls tremors.*

Dementia	A brain disorder that causes severe memory loss and problems thinking.
Demographic information	A person's gender, age, and race. Often asked when a person goes to see a doctor, as part of a **medical history**.
Depression	A condition in which a person feels constant sadness or hopelessness for two weeks or longer. Often includes a lack of energy or motivation to do anything and a lack of interest in activities that used to bring pleasure.
Diagnosis	The issue (usually an illness, condition, or disease) that your doctors believes is causing your **symptoms**.
Dopamine	A chemical in the brain that is often low in people with **Parkinson's disease**.
Dose	The amount of a medicine a person should take (is often listed in milligrams (mg))
Dystonia	A condition that causes stiffness and jerking movements in the muscles.
Electrodes	Wires that have metal contacts on the ends of them that can carry electricity to parts of the brain or body.
Emphysema	A type of **COPD** that causes damage to the lungs making it difficult to breathe.
Essential oil	A concentrated oil made from a plant or flower.
Essential tremor (ET)	A condition, or **movement disorder**, that causes a rhythmic shaking in various parts of the body. Shaking usually occurs when a person's muscles are active (see **action tremor**) or holding against gravity (see **postural tremor**).
ET	See **essential tremor**.
Evaluation	An exam a doctor does to check for medical problems or make sure it is safe for a person to have a surgery.
Family medicine doctor	see **general practitioner**
Focused ultrasound	see **MRI-guided focused ultrasound**
GABA	A chemical made in the brain that may be low in people with **essential tremor**.
Gabapentin	A medicine used to stop seizures that can also help control tremors.
Gamma Knife	A machine that creates a tiny hole in the brain using low-intensity radiation beams to help control tremor.
General exam	see **medical exam**
General practitioner (GP)	A type of doctor who sees both healthy people and people with different kinds of medical problems.
Glioma	The most common type of brain tumor that starts in the brain (is not **metastatic**).
Harmane	A **neurotoxin** that is connected to essential tremor and is found in high levels in the blood of people who eat a lot of meat cooked at high temperatures.

Health chat	*An online event in which a doctor answer questions people submit to a website either in advance or live during a half-hour to one-hour broadcast.*
Health Savings Account	*A type of savings account that some insurance plans offer that lets money be put in (often from a paycheck) without paying tax on it. This money can be used to pay for health and medical bills.*
Heart attack	*Damage to part of the heart that happens suddenly. It is caused by not getting enough blood to parts of the heart, often because of a blood vessel that has a **blood clot**.*
Heart bypass surgery	*A procedure that creates a new path for blood to flow to the part of the heart damaged by a **heart attack**. Also called a "CABG".*
Heart rate	*The number of times per minute the heart beats.*
Hemophilia	*A condition that stops blood from thickening normally when a person has an injury.*
Herb	*A part of a plant that can be used to treat different health problems.*
Herbal medicine	*A type of medicine made from different parts of plants.*
Herbal supplement	see **herbal medicine**
High blood sugar	see **hyperglycemia**
History of present illness (HPI)	*Information taken when a person goes to see a doctor, as part of a **medical** history. It includes the person's current health problem and the reason for seeing the doctor.*
Honeymoon effect	*An effect after **DBS** surgery in which tremors are immediately reduced for a short time, before the DBS system is turned on.*
Hyperglycemia	*A problem in which there is too much sugar in the body, making a person feel sick. Also known as **high blood sugar**. Hyperglycemia over a long time causes many medical problems.*
Hyperthyroidism	*A problem with the **thyroid gland** or with the brain which causes the thyroid hormone levels in the body get too high.*
Hypoglycemia	*A problem in which there is not enough sugar in the body, making it hard for the body to function. Also known as **low blood sugar**. Can also cause seizures.*
Immune system	*A part of the body that helps it fight infections.*
Inderal	*A type of **beta blocker**.*
Infection	*A condition in which a disease, sickness, or poison gets into the body and makes it react.*
Insulin	*A chemical made by the body that controls the amount of blood sugar.*
Intention tremor	*Shaking that happens when a person is aiming for a specific target (e.g., lifting a cup to the mouth). Also known as "action tremor".*
Interaction	*A problem that can happen after a person takes certain different medicines together.*
Internal medicine doctor	see **general practitioner**
Intraoperative MRI suite (IMRIS)	*A room for surgeries in which an **MRI** machine can be slid in and out of the room on ceiling rollers.*

Intravenous line (IV)	*A tube that carries fluids to the body that is inserted through a needle into a vein in the arm, hand, or foot.*
Lesion	*A hole or injury (to the brain).*
Letter of appeal	*A letter a doctor writes to ask an insurance company to cover the cost of a patient's treatment that the insurance company has refused to pay.*
Lidocaine	*A medicine that is injected under the skin to make an area of the body feel less pain.*
Low blood sugar	see *hypoglycemia*
Marijuana	*A medicine that is commonly known as a street drug but has properties that can help treat certain health problems, such as seizures, chronic pain, and tremors.*
Massage therapy	*A treatment in which a therapist gently presses or rubs muscles in the body in order to make tight muscles relax.*
Medical exam	*A procedure in which a doctor checks different parts of the body to find out if the body is working normally or try to figure out what is wrong.*
Medical history	*Information that helps a doctor learn about a person's health and lifestyle. Includes background information, the reason for coming to an appointment, past and current health problems and surgeries, family members' health problems, and other daily behaviors.*
Medical provider	*A doctor or other trained professional who tests for and treats health problems.*
Medical research	*A process in which scientists ask and find answers to health-related questions so that they find out causes of or create new ways to treat diseases and illnesses.*
Meditation	*A practice that involves quieting and clearing the mind and relaxing the body.*
Mediterranean diet	*A set of foods and eating practices often seen in people who live near the Mediterranean Sea. It includes regular meals throughout the day made from fish, poultry, fresh fruits and vegetables, eggs, olive oil, nuts, beans, whole grains, and red wine.*
Mental health	*Psychological, emotional, and social well being.*
Mental status exam	*A test a doctor gives to check a person's knowledge, memory, and awareness.*
Metastasis	*A condition in which a cancer in one part of the body spreads to another part.*
Microelectrode recording (MER)	*A procedure that helps doctors find the best spot in the brain to place a DBS electrode. Involves using many tiny electrodes in the brain to listen to the patterns of sounds different brain cells make.*
Midbrain	*An area in the middle of the brain that helps control seeing, hearing, motion, sleep, and temperature.*
Movement disorder	*An issue that causes problems with normal movement of the body.*

Movement disorder neurologist	*A type of doctor who treats people with problems that affect their ability to move their bodies normally, such as essential tremor, Parkinson's disease, and others.*
MRgFUS	*see MRI-guided focused ultrasound*
MRI	*A machine that takes pictures of the inside of the body using magnets and radio waves. Most helpful to see brain tumors, and other problems with the brain and spinal cord.*
MRI-guided focused ultrasound	*A procedure that creates a tiny hole or **lesion** in the brain using heat from an **ultrasound** to help reduce tremor.*
Multiple sclerosis (MS)	*A condition that causes damage to the brain and spinal cord. It can cause tremors; tingling, numbness, or weakness in the arms or legs; and vision problems.*
Mysoline	*see primidone*
Natural tremor	*see physiologic tremor*
Neuravive	*see MRI-guided focused ultrasound*
Neurological exam	*A procedure a **neurologist** does to check the brain, spinal cord, and nerves. Involves moving the arms and legs, testing strength, sensitivity to touch, reflexes, knowledge, and memory.*
Neurologist	*A doctor who examines and treats people who have problems with their brains, spinal cords, or nerves.*
Neuropsychologist	*A **psychologist** who has special training to work with people who have tremors and problems with their brains, nerves, or spinal cords.*
Neurosurgeon	*A doctor who uses surgery to treat people who have problems with their brains, spinal cords, or nerves.*
Neurotoxin	*A substance that poisons the nerves.*
Nicotine	*The ingredient in cigarettes that makes them habit-forming.*
Occupational therapist	*A **medical professional** who helps people who have an injury, disease, or sickness find ways to keep from getting hurt and to do their regular daily activities.*
Octanoic acid	*A type of alcohol found in foods such as coconut and its products, cow's milk, peanut butter, and palm oil. It can help control tremor and can also be given in pill form as a medicine.*
Pacemaker	*A device implanted in the chest that controls the heart rate.*
Panic attack	*A sudden problem caused by **anxiety** or fear that makes the heart race and a person feel as though they cannot breathe.*
Parasympathetic nervous system	*A system in the body that is active when a person is calm. It relaxes the muscles, slows down breathing, and makes the heart beat slower.*
Parkinson's disease (PD)	*A condition, or **movement disorder**, that often causes shaking in various parts of the body. Shaking usually occurs when a person's muscles are at rest (see **resting tremor**).*
Past surgical history	*Information on any surgery a person has ever had. Asked when a person goes to see a doctor, as part of a **medical history**.*

Patient event	An event held by a doctor, hospital, or company to promote their business to patients who have a specific condition or disease.
PD	See *Parkinson's disease.*
PET scan	A test that uses a special type of radiation to take a picture of the inside of the body. Often helpful to **diagnose Parkinson's disease**.
Physician's assistant (PA)	A **medical professional** who helps doctors during **medical exams** and surgeries.
Physicist	A scientist who studies how things in the world move and interact with one another. Works with a **neurosurgeon** during *Gamma Knife* procedures.
Physiologic tremor	A very fine shaking in the hands and fingers that comes and goes in many people. Also known as **natural tremor**.
Postural tremor	Shaking that happens when a person's muscles are extended and working against gravity (e.g., with arms held out in front of the body.)
Prescription	An order a doctor gives to take a certain medicine or treatment for a health problem.
Primidone	A medicine used to stop seizures that is commonly used to control tremors. A common name for this medicine is Mysoline.
Private practice	The office of a doctor who works independently.
Processed sugar	Sugar, such as table sugar, that is added to food to make it sweeter.
Propranolol	The most common type of **beta blocker**.
Psychologist	A **medical professional** who helps people with issues such as depression, anxiety, and stress by teaching them ways to cope with these problems.
Radiation oncologist	A doctor who is trained to use high-energy radiation to treat cancer and other tumors. Works with a **neurosurgeon** during *Gamma Knife* procedures.
Radiofrequency (RF) ablation	A **surgical** procedure that creates a small hole in the brain using radio waves to help reduce tremor.
RF lesioning	see *radiofrequency ablation*
Reaction	Something that happens to a person after taking a medicine that is not supposed to happen.
Referral	A suggestion from a doctor to see another doctor to help figure out what is wrong.
Repetition (exercise)	One full movement of a specific physical exercise.
Research study	A project in which scientists ask and try to find answers to a specific question by doing different kinds of tests.
Resident	A doctor who is in training to become an expert in an area of medicine.
Resting tremor	Shaking that happens when a person's muscles are at rest (e.g., with hands in a lap).
Review of systems	see *screening questions*

Darlene A Mayo MD FAANS   **STOP SPILLING YOUR SOUP!   The Complete Essential Tremor Solution**

Screening questions	*Asked when a person goes to see a doctor, as part of a **medical history**. A long list of questions about recent or constant problems with different organs of the body.*
SPECT scan	*A test that uses a special type of radiation to take a picture of the inside of the body.*
Social media	*Websites that help people connect with one another and share information.*
Social phobia	*A fear of going out in public places.*
Spinal tap	*A test that involves removing a small amount of fluid from around the spinal cord by placing a needle in the back.*
Stent	*A device that is placed in an artery that is blocked to help blood flow more easily.*
Stereotactic radiosurgery	*see **Gamma Knife***
Stereotactic thalamotomy	*see **radiofrequency ablation***
Stethoscope	*A tool used by medical providers to listen to the heart sounds.*
Stroke	*A sudden problem that damages the brain when an artery carrying blood to the brain gets blocked or when there is bleeding in the brain. It usually makes one side of your body weak or difficult to move and can cause trouble speaking.*
Study	*see **research study***
Substantia nigra	*An area in the bottom of the brain that makes **dopamine**.*
Support groups	*Meetings that help people with a specific issue or disease connect with one another and share information.*
Surgical procedure	*A surgery or operation a person has for a specific issue.*
Surgical technician	*A **medical professional** trained to help with surgery.*
Sympathetic nervous system	*A system in the body that is active when a person is threatened by something. It gives energy to the muscles, more air to the lungs, and makes the heart beat faster.*
Symptom	*A problem with the body or mind's normal functions that is caused by an illness, condition, or disease.*
Tai chi	*A type of Chinese martial art that focuses on smooth, flowing body movements and stretches done in a standing position. It is very easy on the body and joints.*
Thrombectomy	*A surgery to remove a **blood clot** from an artery.*
Thrombolysis	*Dissolving a **blood clot** using special medicines.*
Thyroid	*A small gland in the front of the neck that produces a hormone that affects energy levels, weight, skin, and the brain.*
Topiramate	*A medicine used to stop seizures that can also help control tremors. A common name for this medicine is Topamax.*
Toxin	*A substance that your body makes or that you are exposed to that can be harmful to you.*

Transcranial stimulation (TMS)	*A treatment for tremor and other health problems that involves placing magnets near a person's head. It is thought to work by changing the way brain cells communicate with each other.*
Transfer of care	*When a doctor sends a patient to a different doctor, who knows more about a specific condition or disease, and that doctor takes over treating the patient.*
Treatment plan	*A plan for medical care that a doctor makes for a patient. This may include medicines, **referrals**, or surgery.*
Tremor exam	*A series of tests a doctor gives to find out how severe a tremor is and what makes the tremor worse. It includes checking movements and actions of the patient's arms and legs. This exam helps a doctor find out what is causing a person to shake.*
Tremor severity	*A rating of how badly tremor is affecting a person's life.*
Ultrasound	*A machine that uses sound waves to make pictures of the inside of the body. Can also be used for treatment of tremors in **MRI-guided focused ultrasound.***
Vibration therapy	*A treatment that uses low frequency sound waves delivered to the body often through a special chair that a person sits in during treatment.*
Visualization	*The process of imagining something and seeing a picture of it in the mind.*
Vitamin deficiency	*A condition in which a person does not get enough of a certain vitamin. Can cause many different health problems.*
Weighted utensils	*Spoons, forks, knives with special weights inside their handles that can help people with tremor eat food more easily.*
Whole brain radiation	*A treatment that uses high-energy radiation on the entire brain to treat brain cancer.*
Withdrawal	*A feeling of sickness that happens when a person stops using something habit-forming, such as alcohol, cigarettes, street drugs, and substances such as caffeine.*
X-ray	*A machine that uses a special type of energy to take a picture of the inside of a part of the body.*
Yoga	*A combination of practices, including stretching and strength exercises, breathing techniques, and meditation. Some types focus on holding poses for periods of time in order to build strength, while others focus more on flowing movements.*

Made in United States
North Haven, CT
14 January 2022

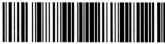